The Intelligent Patient Guide To

Prostate Cancer

The Intelligent Patient Guide To

Prostate Cancer

*All you need to know to take
an active part in your treatment*

S. Larry Goldenberg MD FRCSC

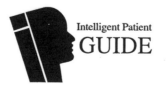

Intelligent Patient
GUIDE

Vancouver, B.C. 1992

Copyright ©1992 by Intelligent Patient Guide Ltd.

Canadian Cataloguing in Publication Data
Goldenberg, S. Larry (Sheldon Larry), 1953-
    The Intelligent Patient Guide to Prostate Cancer

    (The Intelligent Patient Guide Series)
    Includes index.
    ISBN 0-9696125-1-6
    1. Prostate—Cancer—Popular works.
I. Title. II. Series.
RC280.P7G64 1992   616.99'463   C92-091274-5

To obtain a copy of this guide or others in the series, write:

Intelligent Patient Guide Ltd.
320 - 750 West Broadway
Vancouver, British Columbia V5Z 1H4
Canada

Cover design by Fiona MacGregor
Author photograph by Alex Waterhouse-Hayward
Typography by CMY Prepress
Printed in Canada by Friesen Printers

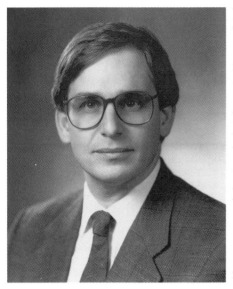

Dr. Goldenberg received his MD from The University of Toronto Medical School and completed surgical training in Urology at the University of British Columbia. He was a Terry Fox research fellow in cancer endocrinology at the British Columbia Cancer Research Centre prior to entering practice.

Dr Goldenberg is a fellow of The Royal College of Surgeons of Canada and diplomate of The American Board of Urology. He is an Associate Professor at The University of British Columbia and staff surgeon at St. Paul's hospital and the British Columbia Cancer Agency in Vancouver.

S. Larry Goldenberg, MD, FRCSC

CONTRIBUTING AUTHORS

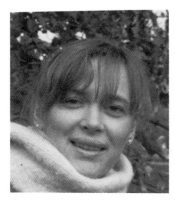

Carolyn Baker, R.N., M.Sc.N.
Clinical Nurse Specialist—Oncology
Vancouver General Hospital

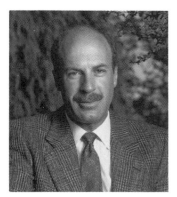

Michael E. Pezim M.D., F.R.C.S.C., D.A.B.S.
Assistant Professor, Department of Surgery, University
of British Columbia. Staff Surgeon, Vancouver General Hospital.
Consultant Surgeon, British Columbia Cancer Agency.

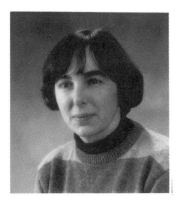

Maria Gyòngyössy Issa Ph.D.
Editor, Intelligent Patient Guide

TABLE OF CONTENTS

Section IX Living with Cancer

Appendix A

Appendix B

Appendix C

Index

THE INTELLIGENT PATIENT GUIDE CONCEPT

We all know friends or loved ones who are battling with or have died of cancer. Yet few people know what cancer really is. Why and how does it start and grow? What does it looks like? How does it kill its host? When a surgeon is forced to abandon an operation and simply close the abdomen in resignation and disgust, what did he see?

The answers to these questions represent only a tiny fraction of a huge range of medical and surgical topics that people read and hear about daily, but have neither the background nor means to interpret correctly. Even bright and otherwise self-sufficient individuals find themselves feeling helpless and frustrated when ill, unable to contribute to their own treatment plan.

IPG believes that the public is capable of understanding many of the complexities of medicine—provided the material is properly presented. The Intelligent Patient Guide series is written for those who want to know more about their illness than can be learned through hurried discussions with a busy physician. It is also for individuals with personalities like ours; experienced and slightly critical people who become distinctly uncomfortable when having to rely totally on someone else's opinion, no matter how much of an expert that person is supposed to be.

You will learn a great deal about malignant disease from this series, but it will not turn you into a cancer surgeon - that would require eight to twelve years of intensive eighteen hour days (and nights). But it will equip you with the basic knowledge required to participate effectively in therapeutic decision-making, will alert you to the situations in which a second opinion is appropriate, and will provide you with some feeling of control in a situation in which patients heretofore felt they had none.

Michael E Pezim MD, FRCSC
Intelligent Patient Guide

For Paula, Adam and Mitchell

SECTION I
WHAT IS A CANCER?

Chapter 1.

What is a Cancer?

TIGHT CONTROL OVER CELL GROWTH

The body's growth is the result of both the enlargement of individual **cells**, and an increase of their total number (fig 1). Cells increase in number through a process called **mitosis** (cell division). A cell divides into two identical **daughter cells**. If cell division were to occur too often, the body would grow inordinately. Conversely, too few cell divisions would result in a breakdown of body parts as worn-out cells went unreplaced. To prevent the consequences of either excessive or inadequate numbers of cell divisions, *the body maintains tight control* over the rate of growth and division of each of its billions of cells.

At times, some overproduction is required. A callous on the foot is an overproduction of skin cells required for protection against the repeated trauma of an abrasive shoe. However, in this instance the body remains in complete control — when the offending stimulus is removed, the callous disappears.

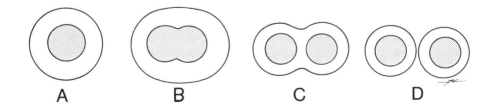

A   B   C   D

Figure 1

1

Rates of cell growth vary from one part of the body to another. Cells lining the intestine have a short life span and consequently have one of the highest rates of growth and replacement in the body. The entire intestinal lining is replaced every 3 days. The cells of the brain are quite different, they do not increase in numbers at all following early childhood, and there is no mechanism available for the replacement of lost cells. Hence, most brain injuries are unfortunately permanent. The heart is another organ in which cell division is limited, and its ability to repair itself following a heart attack is imperfect.

Interestingly, the rate of cancer development in an organ seems to relate directly to the rate of cell divisions within that organ. The skin and intestine, areas of high rates of cell division and turnover, are organs in which cancer is relatively common. Cancers of the brain and heart are extremely rare.

SANCTITY OF THE GENE PACKAGE

Cells of similar appearance and function are grouped together as a team, working as a unit to accomplish a particular task. Such cell groups are known as **organs**. The liver is an organ consisting of millions of liver cells, each similar in appearance and function to its neighboring liver cell.

Although the cells of one organ may differ tremendously in appearance and function from those of another organ (*eg* liver *versus* kidney), all cells of the body have one thing in common: they contain an identical set of **genes**. Genes contain the directions for the function and behavior of the cell, and act as the cell's 'instruction manual.'

A liver cell behaves like a liver cell *not* because it contains genes that are different from those of an intestinal cell, but because it takes its instructions only from the liver 'chapter' of the genetic instruction manual. Even though all cells have a complete and identical set of genes, each cell follows a pattern of growth, division and function characteristic of the organ within which it resides.

At one time each of us consisted of only one cell, a fertilized egg cell. That cell had to contain the complete information required for the development of a complete human. The unique gene package contained within that single cell was a product of the combination of the two *half-sets* of genes carried by the egg and sperm of our parents. (Incidentally, egg and sperm cells are the only cells permitted to carry half-sets of genes.) Division of that original cell and countless further divisions eventually developed into a human being.

During the process of cell division, *an exact duplicate* of the gene package is made just before the cell divides into two daughter cells. In this way, each daughter cell receives a complete and identical copy of the parent cell's gene package. Thus, every cell of an 80 year-old person contains an identical duplication of the gene package that was created in the initial fertilization process some 80 years and 9 months earlier!

THE CLONE THEORY OF CANCER DEVELOPMENT

Despite the incredible accuracy with which cells duplicate, gene duplication errors do occur, creating daughter cells with changed, abnormal gene packages (fig 2). For example, a daughter cell may receive half of a particular strand of genes instead of the full strand, leaving it without a portion of instructions. The other daughter cell receives the extra genetic material, thus resulting in two abnormal cells. These changed, abnormal cells are known as **mutant cells**

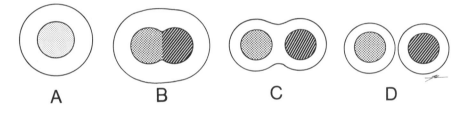

A   B   C   D

Figure 2

Fortunately, the vast majority of mutant cells are incapable of surviving, or are destroyed by the body's **immune system**. If, however, the change is such that the mutant cell possesses both the capabilities for survival and an ability to hide from the the immune system, it may begin to divide into identical *mutant daughter cells*. In this way, the progeny of the mutant daughter cell, a **clone** of mutant cells, is established within the body. All cells of the clone are identical by virtue of possessing a gene package that is unique to them, but different from the normal cells of the body. Suddenly, the body is harbouring a new line of cells (**mutant clone**), that it cannot destroy (fig 3).

In some cases, the mutant clone of cells will behave in a harmless fashion, remaining small and localized. This type of clone is commonly called a **benign neoplasm**: benign meaning 'harmless' and neoplasm meaning 'new growth.' Benign neoplasms may develop in any part of the body, and may include harmless breast lumps, skin abnormalities, and small polyps arising within the lining of the intestine.

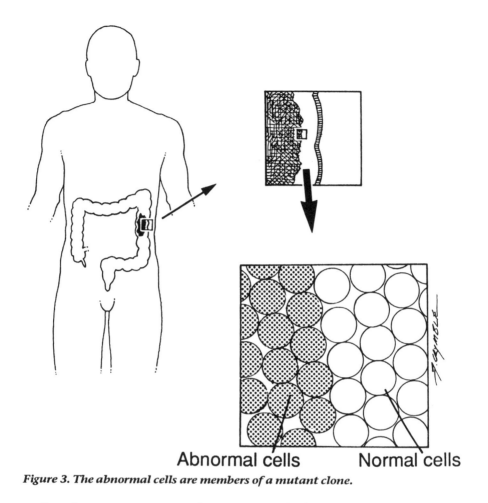

Abnormal cells   **Normal cells**

Figure 3. The abnormal cells are members of a mutant clone.

In other cases, a mutant clone may evade the mechanisms that exist to control cell growth and divide with complete disregard for the needs or limitations of the body. Such cells may grow through the organs in which they reside or spread as tiny cell clumps through the bloodstream to other organs where they become implanted, grow into a mass and eventually overwhelm and destroy that organ. A clone of cells that pursues this aggressive behavior is called a **malignant neoplasm**. More commonly, it is called a **cancer**.

Chapter 2
The Unique Abilities of the Cancer Cell

The power of the cancer cell lies in its disregard for the basic principles of cell growth and division, and its ability to defeat the body's immune system.

UNCONTROLLED GROWTH

Under normal conditions, the rate of cell growth and division is subject to strict control by the body. If this were not the case, there would be nothing to prevent one arm from growing longer than the other, or the brain from growing too large for the skull. Cell growth and division rates are set out in the gene package that each cell is programmed to read, and are modified by signals within the body.

Cancer cells defy the body's regulations regarding controlled growth by enlarging and dividing at their own, usually much faster pace, unencumbered by the constraints placed on their neighboring normal cells. As the number of cancer cells in a small area increase, a lump, or **tumor**, is formed.

Cancer cells have the ability to stimulate the development of blood vessels to supply them with nutrients. A cancer's ability to increase its blood supply not only enhances its own growth, but may lead to a relative 'drought' of bloodstream nutrients and oxygen for surrounding normal cells, impairing their ability to function properly. Occasionally, a cancer's wild growth rate backfires. The cancer may grow so rapidly that it almost destroys itself by enlarging faster than its feeding vessels can deliver oxygen. When this happens, part of the cancer may suddenly die. This death of a group of cells within a cancer is known as **necrosis**.

ABILITY TO SPREAD

The second basic principle governing most normal cells is that they remain in the area in which they belong, and do not spread to other parts of the body. Cancer cells disregard this principle and may disseminate throughout the body in several ways.

5

Into Adjacent Organs

Cancer cells may grow right through the confines of the organ in which they develop (fig 4A). Thus, a cancer of the pancreas may **invade** (grow into) the adjacent intestine. The patient would have abdominal pain from blockage of the bowel at that level.

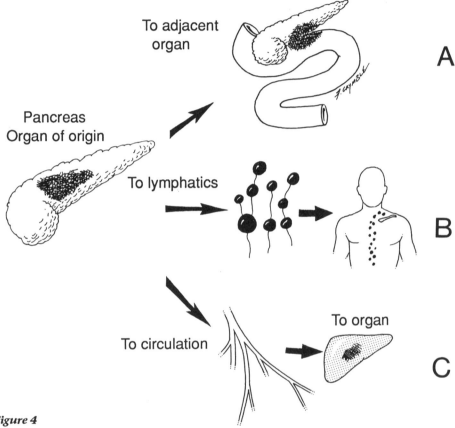

To adjacent organ

Pancreas Organ of origin

To lymphatics

To circulation

To organ

A

B

C

Figure 4

Into Lymph Nodes

Tissue fluid is produced in most areas of the body as part of normal function. The fluid travels along **lymphatic vessels**, small transparent conduits that look like tiny, bloodless veins, and eventually finds its way into the bloodstream. **Lymph nodes** are small lima bean-shaped structures located at various points along the lymphatic vessels. We occasionally become aware of the presence of lymph nodes when an area of our body becomes inflamed or injured, causing the nodes to become enlarged. Lymph nodes are the structures that the doctor feels under the jaw when someone has a throat infection. They are sometimes mistakenly referred to as 'swollen glands.' Cancer cells may spread to the lymph nodes by the lymphatic vessels (fig 4B). Once in the lymph node, the cancer cells may implant themselves and begin growing and dividing into a cancerous mass. Such a lymph node is said to be **'involved'** with cancer.

To Distant Organs

An established cancer may spread to other, quite distant organs of the body, multiplying its destructive effects (fig 4C). This type of spread occurs by way of the blood as it is pumped along in the circulatory system. As a cancer grows at its **primary site** (original site), some of the cancer cells may break off and get swept away in the blood as it makes its way back to the lungs for reoxygenation. Occasionally, these floating clumps of cancer cells will become lodged in one of the organs that the blood passes through. If they lodge at a site that provides the right conditions for growth, they may begin growing and dividing to form a new cancer mass.

This new group of cancer cells, growing somewhere other than the primary site, is known as a **metastasis** or **secondary site**.

ABILITY TO DEFY THE IMMUNE SYSTEM

The **immune system** consists of a group of highly-sophisticated cells specialized to recognize and destroy 'foreign' material such as bacteria, viruses, fungi and unfamiliar cells. The immune system's weapons include 'killer cells' and antibodies. Killer cells attack alien cells directly. Antibodies are proteins that act like mines — they attach themselves to the intruder and stimulate the release of highly toxic materials which lead to the destruction of the intruder. Both killer cells and antibodies are produced by the immune system.

By means of the blood and lymphatic circulations, the immune system's 'detective' cells are constantly being carried throughout the body, providing early recognition of foreign substances (fig 5). The bloodstream also serves to transport vast numbers of antibodies and killer white blood cells to the 'battlefield' once an intruder has been identified.

How does the immune system know what belongs and what does not? At some point during the growth of the human fetus, the immune system takes an 'inventory' in which all cells and substances currently in the body are accepted as being genuine components of the body. They belong: they are labelled as 'self.' As the immune system grows in sophistication towards the point of birth, it develops the means to become activated toward any substance that has not been itemized in the inventory.

One of the roles of the immune system of the body is to identify and destroy the mutant cells that result from an error in cell division, mutant cells that could otherwise result in the beginnings of a cancer. In order for a mutant cell to survive, it must somehow avoid identification and destruction by the immune system.

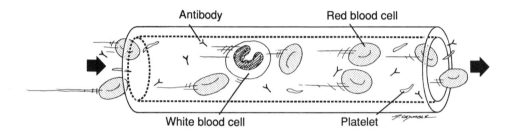

Figure 5. Some of the important constituents of blood travelling within a blood vessel.

Chapter 3

How Does Cancer Kill?

Cancer kills its 'host' through complications of uncontrolled growth at the original (primary) site of its development, or through widespread damage to the body from spread to other organs (metastases).

DEATH THROUGH UNRESTRAINED GROWTH AT THE PRIMARY SITE

Unrestrained growth of a cancer at the primary site may harm the host simply by its sheer size. A cancer in the colon will eventually become large enough to block off the bowel completely. A cancer of the prostate may grow large enough to block the flow of urine from the kidneys. Both situations are lethal unless treated by emergency surgery.

The effects of a cancer growing within the brain are even more devastating because brain tissue is so soft and easily compressed. As a brain cancer grows, the surrounding normal brain becomes squeezed between the cancer and the inside of the skull, leading to seizures and severe brain dysfunction which, when it impairs essential functions such as control of breathing or heart-beat, can cause death.

Death may also come by invasion of the cancer into a neighboring body part. The most dramatic example of this is the penetration of a major blood vessel by an adjacent cancer, leading to a sudden massive **hemorrhage**.

DEATH BY METASTASES

Many people who die of cancer do so as a result of the effects of **metastases**, new colonies of cancer cells that have travelled to and taken up residence in other parts of the body. Metastases are sometimes called **secondaries**. It is this ability to spread that makes cancer such a formidable opponent. Growing metastases eventually destroy the organs in which they reside (fig 6), and that can lead to death.

9

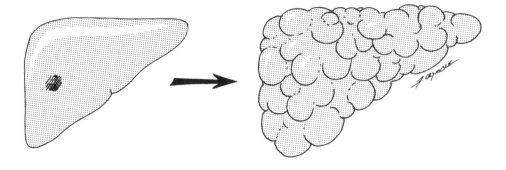

Figure 6. As metastases grow within the liver they destroy the normal tissue and lead to liver failure.

Metastases in organs far from the original site of cancer growth are the result of clumps of cancer cells breaking away from the main cancer and floating off in the bloodstream. Some of the more common locations for metastases are the liver, lung, brain and bone. Metastatic colonies of cancer cells in the liver lead to an inability of the liver to detoxify blood or to regulate body protein and glucose metabolism. Metastases in the lungs will gradually reduce the lungs' ability to transfer oxygen to the blood. Brain metastases lead to compression and destruction of normal brain tissue. Bone metastases may result in bone pain or sudden fractures.

Chapter 4
The Multiple Personalities of Cancer

There are many different types of cancers. Each type is distinguished by the cells in which the cancer originates. Thus, a cancer may arise from cells lining ducts or glands, muscle cells, nerve cells or fat cells. Each of these cancers behaves differently and is called by a different name: **adenocarcinoma** (cancer of the lining cells), **leiomyosarcoma** (cancer of the muscle cells), **neurosarcoma** (cancer of the nerve cells) and **liposarcoma** (cancer of the fat cells). Thus, if a person has a cancer, it is important to know what type of cancer it is to predict how it will behave and how best to treat it.

THE SAME TYPE OF CANCER MAY VARY IN AGGRESSIVENESS

The picture is further complicated by the fact that cancers of similar cell types may vary in aggressiveness from one case to another. In one person an adenocarcinoma may remain small and localized, while in another it may be widespread by the time it is identified.

A cancer's aggressiveness can be determined by establishing how far it has already spread (**staging** the cancer), and by assessing the appearance of individual cells under the microscope (**grading** the cancer). This information helps the physician plan the most appropriate therapy and provides information regarding **prognosis** (likelihood of cure).

STAGING THE CANCER: HAS IT SPREAD?

When a cancer is first identified, the physician attempts to take a 'snapshot' of how far it has spread. By asking questions, examining the patient thoroughly and applying a variety of tests, he or she aims to **stage** the cancer.

In some cases, the staging process may be relatively simple. For a patient with cancer and an enlarged, irregular liver caused by multiple metastases, a physician may be able to tell by touch alone that the cancer is in an advanced stage, having already spread to the liver.

Alternatively, careful questioning and physical examination may fail to show that the cancer has spread beyond its primary site, which could mean that it is at an early-stage, and remains localized. Laboratory investigations and special studies are ordered to rule out the presence of metastases and to confirm the early stage of the cancer. In some instances, unfortunately, very sensitive staging studies reveal metastases which are too small to be detected by simple physical examination.

GRADING THE CANCER: HOW ABNORMAL ARE THE CELLS?

The **grade** of a cancer is an assessment of cell appearance assigned by a **pathologist**, a physician who specializes in the microscopic evaluation of disease. At some time before or during treatment of a cancer, the treating physician will obtain a sample of the cancer (**biopsy**) for the pathologist to view under the microscope. The pathologist will assign the cancer a grade based on its microscopic appearance.

Cells of a cancer are identified microscopically based on a variety of features that distinguish them from normal cells. Such characteristics include cell size, shape, uniformity or the ability to stain certain colors when dyes are placed on them. *The grade of a cancer is based on the degree to which its cells deviate from normal cells of that organ,* the greater the difference, the higher the grade. **High-grade cancers** grow rapidly and metastasize early. **Low-grade cancers** are less aggressive and may grow slowly without metastasizing for long periods. A number of interchangeable terms are used by physicians to describe the grade of a cancer (**see HIGHLIGHT on Grading Terminology Quagmire**).

HOW STAGE AND GRADE INFORMATION ARE USED

When dealing with people who have cancer, the physician tries at best to **cure** them, and at least to **palliate** them. Palliation means a treatment that aims to reduce suffering from cancer symptoms, but which is not expected to provide a cure.

Cancers that are in an **early stage** (localized to one area) are the most easily cured. Treatment is usually a matter of removing or destroying that area. A cancer that is both low-grade *and* at an early stage represents the most favorable situation: a not-too-aggressive cancer that has yet to spread.

Alternatively, if staging tests reveal that the cancer has spread to distant parts of the body (**late-stage**), cure may not be possible. If the person has few symptoms, it may be best to reserve any potentially noxious palliative treatment until the appearance of significant symptoms (pain, bleeding) justifies such treatment. In other cases, palliation may best be achieved by early surgery, radiotherapy or chemotherapy in the hope of lengthening the symptom-free period. Complex treatment decisions such as this must be made individually. For the patient and the family, making an appropriate decision requires the input of an experienced and compassionate team of cancer specialists.

Especially challenging situations are faced when a late-stage cancer is of low grade, or a high-grade cancer is found at an early stage. In the case of a late-stage cancer of low grade, the surgeon will sometimes attempt major surgery to remove the primary site as well as metastases in the liver, lungs or other parts of the body, hoping that the cancer is still curable because of its

Grading Terminology Quagmire

There are a confusing variety of terms used to designate grade. The simplest is the high/low system in which a microscopically nasty-looking cancer is called **high-grade** cancer while a less nasty-looking cancer is called a **low-grade** cancer. A cancer of intermediate appearance is called an **average-grade** cancer.

Another system of grading is named after an American pathologist named Broder. **Broder's** labels a nasty-looking cancer as a grade 4 cancer, while an average-looking cancer is a grade 2 or 3.

The most commonly used system is the **differentiation system**. This one is a bit hard to describe. It is based on the understanding that a *normal* cell is a 'differentiated' cell. Differentiated from what? Differentiated from the original cells of a human embryo. Embryo cells have not yet differentiated into the various cell types of the body (liver cells, muscle cells, etc.) and therefore had a particular appearance - an undifferentiated appearance. As we grow from an embryo, our cells differentiate

(become different) from the original cells and develop into the cells of our various organs. Microscopically, cancer cells appear more similar to those embryonal cells than to normal, differentiated cells. A cancer made up of **poorly-differentiated** cells is one which has cells that appear like original embryo cells and very much unlike normal adult cells. Because it is so different from what a normal cell is supposed to look like, the poorly-differentiated cancer is a bad actor. It has not differentiated enough to develop manners and to comply with the rules and regulations of the body. A cancer made up of poorly-differentiated cells is therefore a high-grade (nasty) cancer. A **well-differentiated** cancer is low-grade (better). An average-grade cancer in the differentiation system is a **moderately-differentiated** or **moderately-well-differentiated** cancer.

Another word that you might hear is **anaplastic**. Anaplastic means very-poorly differentiated - a high-grade (nasty) cancer.

13

low grade. This 'going for broke' plan is an option, provided the patient understands the risks and aims of the treatment and is physically (and mentally) capable of undergoing what needs to be done. The opposite combination of an early stage but high-grade cancer will frequently frustrate any attempt to cure what appears to be only a localized problem. High-grade cancers tend to recur or appear as metastases following even the most complete and apparently successful operation.

TABLE 1. — CANCER GRADE: VARIOUS TERMINOLOGIES

least aggressive	average	most aggressive
low-grade	medium-grade	high-grade
Broder's 1	Broder's 2, 3	Broder's 4
well-differentiated	moderately-well differentiated	poorly-differentiated anaplastic
Gleason 2, 3, 4	Gleason (4),5, 6, 7	Gleason 8, 9, 10

SECTION II:
THE PROSTATE GLAND

Chapter 5

What is the Prostate Gland?

The **prostate gland** is part of the urinary and reproductive systems of the male; women do not have a prostate gland. The prostate lies just below the urinary bladder at the base of the penis, directly in front of the lower rectum (figs 7 & 8). In a normal, young man it is the size of a walnut, but with age and continuous exposure to the male sex hormone **testosterone**, the gland grows larger.

Sperm from the testicles ascend *via* the **vas deferens** through the groin, the prostate gland and the **ejaculatory ducts** into the **urethra**. The ejaculatory ducts are also connected to the **seminal vesicles**, sperm-storing containers, which lie directly behind the prostate and the lower bladder. The seminal vesicles are considered to be an extension of the prostate gland.

The top of the prostate is attached directly to the **bladder**. The urethra courses through the prostate gland and ends at the tip of the penis. The prostate surrounds the passageway for the normal flow of urine and, in its walls along the urethra, has muscle fibers that assist urinary control. It also produces **ejaculatory fluid**, which contains proteins and minerals that maintain the sperm needed for reproduction. It is estimated that 80% of the fluid released during ejaculation is produced by the prostate gland.

This intimate anatomical relationship between the prostate and other organs within the pelvis means that problems originating in the prostate may cause abnormal sensations anywhere in the lower abdomen or lower back, penis, rectum or scrotum.

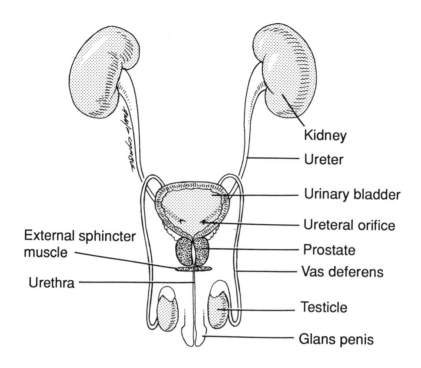

Kidney

Ureter

Urinary bladder

Ureteral orifice

External sphincter muscle

Prostate

Urethra

Vas deferens

Testicle

Glans penis

Figure 7. Frontal view

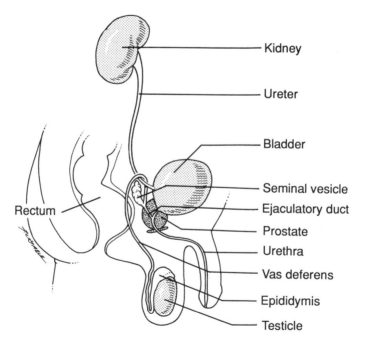

Kidney

Ureter

Bladder

Seminal vesicle

Rectum

Ejaculatory duct

Prostate

Urethra

Vas deferens

Epididymis

Testicle

Figure 8. Side view

16

Chapter 6
Diseases of the Prostate

The prostate gland is susceptible to three common diseases: prostatitis, benign prostatic hyperplasia (BPH), and cancer.

PROSTATITIS

Men of any age can develop a prostate infection called **prostatitis**. Prostatitis can be acquired though sexual contact, but often it develops for no apparent reason. Prostatitis may be acute (sudden, severe and transient) or chronic (slow to develop but persistent).

Acute Prostatitis

Acute prostatitis causes severe, sudden symptoms: a strong and frequent urge to pass urine, burning urination, and difficulty getting the urine to pass. Fortunately, acute prostatitis can be completely cured with appropriate medical treatment that includes antibiotics, anti-inflammatory drugs, bed rest, and plenty of fluids.

Chronic Prostatitis

Chronic prostatitis has a slower onset than acute prostatitis and its symptoms are more annoying than dangerous. A man with this condition will complain of frequent and strong urges to urinate ('frequency' and 'urgency'); some slowing of the stream; and an ache or pain in the genitals, rectum, lower abdomen or lower back. Treatment of chronic prostatitis includes long-term antibiotics, anti-inflammatory drugs, zinc supplements, frequent ejaculations ('do your homework'), and avoidance of caffeine, alcohol, spicy foods, and smoking, all of which are known irritants of the urinary tract.

BENIGN PROSTATIC HYPERPLASIA

As a man gets older, his prostate enlarges. This condition is called **benign prostatic hyperplasia** (meaning benign excess growth) or **BPH**. The enlarged prostate impinges on the urethra and begins to obstruct the flow of urine from the bladder (fig 9). As this occurs, the bladder, which is a muscular sac,

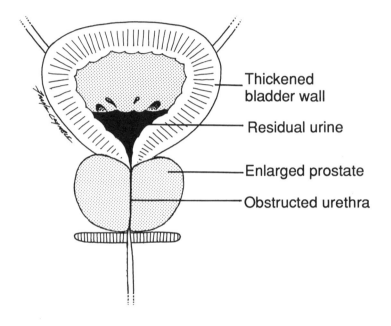

Thickened bladder wall

Residual urine

Enlarged prostate

Obstructed urethra

Figure 9

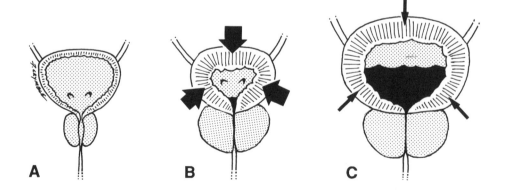

A   B   C

Figure 10

18

compensates by becoming thicker and stronger and contracting harder to overcome the obstruction (fig 10B). Ultimately, however, the urethra may become so narrow that the bladder is unable to mount enough pressure to empty completely. Incomplete emptying permits 'residual urine' to remain in the bladder after voiding (fig 10C). Because the residual urine takes up space, the bladder will be full again that much sooner, which causes more frequent urinations (fig 11). When the full-blown syndrome (sometimes called **prostatism**) is present, the individual will notice a weakness of the urine stream, a need to strain to maximize emptying, a sense of incomplete emptying of the bladder, and an increased frequency of urination.

Occasionally, an enlarged prostate can bleed into the urine ('**hematuria**'). Such bleeding is usually painless. It happens because small, fragile blood vessels on the prostate surface stretch and rupture, usually due to the pressure of straining: straining to urinate, or from lifting or crouching. In most cases the blood can only be seen under a microscope. It is rare for anyone to lose a significant amount of blood from a small vessel on the prostate gland. If blood in the urine is noticed, however, it should prompt a visit to the urologist to rule out other possible (and more serious) causes of hematuria such as growths on the bladder wall or in the kidney.

Almost all men with normally functioning testicles eventually develop **BPH**. The incidence is so high that a 50 year-old man has a 50:50 chance of suffering the consequences of a blocked urinary channel and requiring medical or surgical intervention.

CANCER

Unlike benign hyperplasia in which the excess growth is confined to the gland, a cancer is characterized by uncontrolled cell division of abnormal cells which can replace much of the prostate and spread to other parts of the body. Both BPH and cancer are influenced by the presence of the male hormone testosterone and both are extremely common. In fact, both are so common that a man can have both diseases just as a matter of (bad) luck. However, there is no evidence to suggest that BPH leads to cancer.

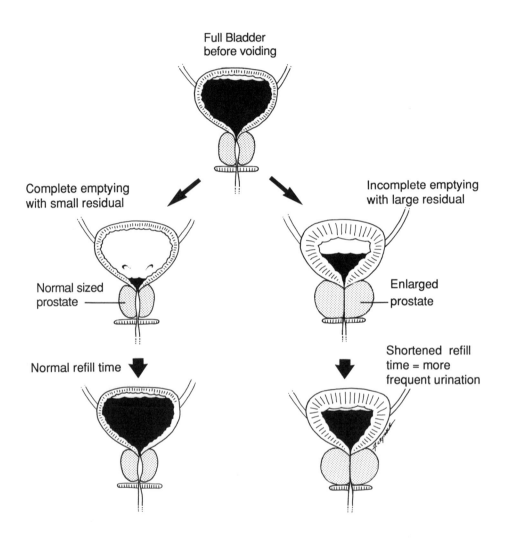

Full Bladder
before voiding

Complete emptying
with small residual

Incomplete emptying
with large residual

Normal sized
prostate

Enlarged
prostate

Normal refill time

Shortened refill
time = more
frequent urination

Figure 11

20

SECTION III: THE SCOPE OF THE PROSTATE CANCER PROBLEM

Chapter 7

How Common is Prostate Cancer?

CANCER IN GENERAL

Cancer is the second most common cause of adult deaths, following heart disease, and is the first or second leading cause of death in all age groups. Of the more than two million deaths each year in the United States, 460,000 (23%) are from cancer.

Over one million new cases of cancer were diagnosed in the United States in 1991, and just over half that number of patients will die of the disease. The estimated number of new cases in Canada during the same period is 100,000. For each new case of cancer at least a dozen people—relatives, friends, business associates, *etc.* will be affected by the person's illness.

Over half of the new cancer cases and deaths are caused by the three most frequent types of cancer. For men, these are cancer of the lung, prostate gland and colorectum; for women, breast, lung and colorectum. Statistical trends suggest that for men, the numbers of lung and prostate cancer are on the increase, while colon and rectal cancer numbers are stable. For women, the picture is different; while lung cancer is increasing for them too, breast cancer numbers are stable and colorectal cancer is actually decreasing.

PROSTATE CANCER SPECIFICALLY

The global incidence of prostate cancer has risen dramatically in the past 20 years. In 1970 the **incidence** was 33 cases per 100,000 males but by 1991 the incidence had increased to 56 cases per 100,000 (an increase of 63%). Today, prostate cancer is the most common cancer that affects the North American male, accounting for 20% (106,000) of all newly diagnosed cancers. In 1991, it caused 11% of male cancer deaths (30,000), equaling colorectal cancer. The number of prostate cancer cases is projected to increase by 65% in the decade 1991 to 2001 and will be numerically second only to breast cancer. It is estimated that a North American male born today has a 9% chance of being diagnosed with prostate cancer during his life-time and a 3% chance of dying from the disease.

The increased incidence of prostate cancer during the past two decades is due to several factors. First, men live longer and are therefore at risk for a longer period of time. Second, family physicians do more digital rectal examinations because of a greater understanding of the prevalence of prostate problems. Finally, early detection tools such as **serum tumor markers**, and **transrectal ultrasound** are becoming more widely used (Chapter 13 and Chapter 14). Thus, part of the increase of prostate cancer may be explained by improved methods used to detect it. Better detection of prostate cancer can translate into an *apparent* increased incidence because this disease is often slow-growing and 'occult,' and in many cases the patients die of other problems before the prostate disease can have its impact. In the past, such individuals would not have been diagnosed as having prostate cancer except perhaps by autopsy. In other cancers, such as lung cancer, a better means of diagnosis would not affect incidence figures because lung cancer is so aggressive that almost everyone who develops it manifests symptoms sooner or later.

Prostate cancer is unusual for men under the age of 40 but it becomes increasingly common with advancing age. Most cases (95%) are diagnosed in men between 45 and 89 years, with an average age of 70 at diagnosis. Unfortunately, in nearly 40% of the cases the cancer is extensive by the time the disease is detected. These men with advanced cancer are considered incurable even though they may survive several years and have a reasonable quality of life most of that time. Only 60% of prostate cancers are discovered when they are still localized within the prostate gland and are potentially curable by aggressive therapy.

Given the relationship between age and prostate diseases, it becomes clear that as the male life span increases, there will be an escalating burden on society to provide medical care for prostate cancer. To date, there is no evidence that any specific environmental or dietary factors have increased the incidence of prostate cancer. Until there is a better understanding of why prostate cancer develops, it is essential to discover methods of early diagnosis and control in order to reduce suffering and death from this disease.

Chapter 8
Prostate Cancer Pathology

ADENOCARCINOMA

The prostate gland (fig 12) is made up of thousands of small, fluid-producing **glands** interspersed with a muscular framework of supporting tissues, fibrous cells, blood vessels and nerves. The most common prostate cancer is the type that develops within the glands themselves and is called an **adenocarcinoma**, 'adeno' meaning gland and 'carcinoma' being another term for cancer. Adenocarcinomas start as a single cell then grow out to involve the rest of the prostate. They can spread beyond the prostate to adjacent or distant tissues.

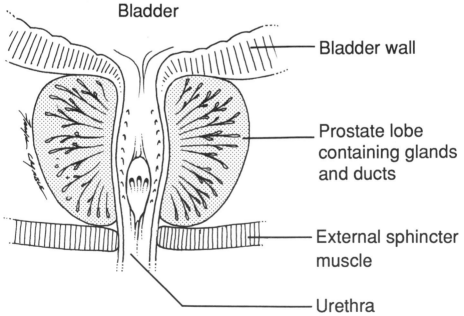

Bladder

Bladder wall

Prostate lobe containing glands and ducts

External sphincter muscle

Urethra

Figure 12. The prostate contains many glands and ducts.

Most cases of prostate cancer are detected by a careful **digital rectal examination** of the gland during a routine medical examination. A physician can assess the extent of the cancer and determine whether or not it is limited to the tissues of the gland or has spread to adjacent tissues.

Cancer that originates within the confines of the prostate will grow slowly, eventually growing into the surrounding tissues. As it impinges on the urethra it will slow the urine stream, cause a feeling of urgency to urinate or an increased frequency of urination (as occurs in BPH; see fig 11). The growing cancer may rupture blood vessels in the lining tissue of the urinary channel, causing variable degrees of **hematuria** (blood in the urine). If it grows large enough to block both of the **ureters** (channels which lead from the kidneys into the bladder), kidney failure may result (fig 13). This complication can be fatal if not treated quickly (Chapter 30).

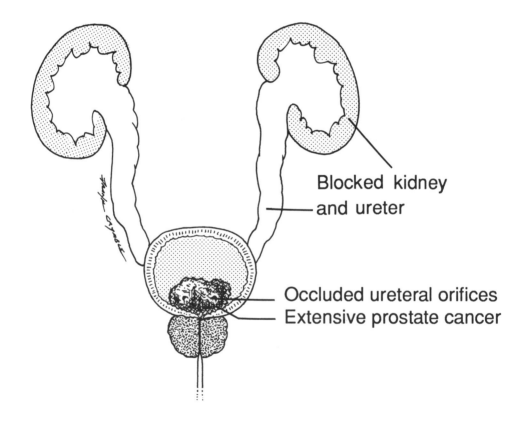

Blocked kidney and ureter

Occluded ureteral orifices
Extensive prostate cancer

Figure 13. Prostate cancer blocking both ureters.

Prostate cancer may be carried by the blood or lymphatic systems and spread (**metastasize**) to other parts of the body, particularly to the bones. In extreme cases, the cancer may damage so much of the bone marrow that there is not enough marrow to produce red and white blood cells. A lack of red cells results in **anemia** while a lack of white cells reduces the body's ability to fight infection. At late stages, prostate cancer may spread to other organs such as the lung, liver or the brain.

Life-expectancy depends on the amount of cancer already present when it is discovered, the type of treatment chosen, and the response of the cancer and the patient to treatment. In its *earliest* stages, prostate cancer may not shorten overall life-expectancy. This is because the cancer grows slowly and is mostly found in older men who often have other illnesses such as heart disease or diabetes. At *later* stages of cancer, life-expectancy may range from 6 months to 10 years or more, with the average duration of life being approximately 24 months after the disease is first detected and treated.

OTHER CANCERS OF THE PROSTATE

Adenocarcinoma is by far the most common type of prostate cancer. However, there are a few *exceedingly rare types* of prostate cancer that are mentioned here for the sake of completeness. A **transitional cell carcinoma,** a cancer more commonly found in the bladder, may originate in the lining cells of the urine channel and grow down into the prostate gland. Less commonly, a transitional cell cancer will arise within the prostate itself where it is usually very aggressive and is often already beyond cure when it is diagnosed. An **endometrioid cancer** arises from female-type cells which remain in the prostate gland from the time of embryonic development. Rare cancers called **sarcomas** can involve the prostate, as well as the bladder and other pelvic organs, but more often occur in young children.

Chapter 9

What Causes Prostate Cancer?

It is not yet clear why prostate cancer develops, but experimental and population-based studies provide insight into the factors that may play a role.

AGE

Prostate cancer has a definite link to age. Eighty percent of prostate cancers are diagnosed in men over 65 years, and only 1% are found in men younger than 50 years.

HORMONES

It is postulated that the reason advanced age may be so important a risk factor is because of the long-term exposure of the prostate cells to the male hormone **testosterone**. Testosterone is the hormone responsible for the development of male sexual characteristics at puberty, including **libido** (sex drive), body hair, beard, deepening voice and genital enlargement. After puberty, testosterone is produced continuously by the testicles and circulates in the bloodstream. It also stimulates the prostate to grow and, particularly in men over 40, to develop BPH as well as cancerous growths.

GENETIC, GEOGRAPHIC AND ENVIRONMENTAL FACTORS

There are striking differences in the incidence of prostate cancer on a worldwide basis and even among ethnic groups within the same area. For example, there is a 120-fold difference between the group with the highest incidence (black American men) and the lowest (men from Shanghai, China). As well, black American men have double the mortality or death rate compared to that of white Americans. Statistics also reveal that among white men in general, prostate cancer has the highest death rate for Scandinavians.

The reasons for these differences are not known.

Some studies have found that men with an affected close relative, such as a father or brother, may be twice as likely to develop prostate cancer as men with no affected relatives. Despite these data, it is still unclear whether prostate cancer is caused by either hereditary or environmental factors.

Some cancers, such as those of the colorectum and breast, have been linked to a high intake of **dietary fat**. While most available data do show an association between fat intake and prostate cancer, further study is necessary to establish whether this is an important relationship.

Smoking and **alcohol** consumption do not seem to increase the likelihood of developing prostate cancer. There is conflicting evidence of a link between workplace **cadmium** exposure, used in welding, electroplating, and alkaline battery industries, and predisposition to an earlier development of prostate cancer.

SEXUAL AND PHYSICAL ACTIVITY

The evidence that sexual experience or venereal diseases put a man at risk for prostate cancer is not convincing. Equal numbers of scientific studies stand for and against such an association. Similarly, there is no correlation between physical exercise and the development of prostate disease. While there is ongoing controversy as to whether **vasectomy** is a risk factor for the development of prostate cancer, the majority of evidence suggests that there is no relationship.

Chapter 10
Prevention - Is It Possible?

Currently, there are no practical means of preventing prostate cancer. Scientists are still unable to link its causes to any environmental, dietary, or drug agent. They have also *ruled out* the association between cancer of the prostate and benign BPH tumors, previous infection of the prostate, age at the start or frequency of sexual activity, anal intercourse, exercise, hygiene, or the presence of genital cancers in a sexual partner.

Compelling evidence does exist, however, that testosterone stimulates prostate cells to grow and that with time some of these cells escape normal control mechanisms and become malignant. Thus, the only absolute means of preventing prostate cancer is to castrate all males before puberty! Obviously, that is not a measure likely to catch on. It is interesting to note, however, that **castration** has been used throughout history as an instrument of punishment and as a way of guaranteeing a supply of male sopranos or of eunuchs for guard duty in harems. As far as we know, prostate cancer has never been known to develop in a male who was castrated before puberty (**eunuch**).

There is scientific evidence to support the fact that **zinc** is an important mineral for prostate tissue, and that zinc supplements may fight prostate disease. This may be true for prostatitis, but there is no evidence that zinc prevents other prostate diseases, including cancer. Other natural remedies recommended by nutritionists include pumpkin seeds, bee pollen, and cold-pressed vegetable oil, none of which have been shown scientifically to be of any preventative value, but are certainly not harmful in moderation.

A common fear is that a man with prostate cancer may cause his sexual partner to develop a cancer of the sex organs. This is absolutely impossible and this misconception should not interfere with a cancer patient's physical relationships before, during, or after treatment. It is also clear that **celibacy** *does not* prevent the development of prostate cancer.

28

SECTION IV: DETECTION

Chapter 11

Symptoms and Signs

A cancer may declare its presence by giving rise to **symptoms** that the patient can describe to the doctor, or it may produce physical **signs** that the physician can detect during a physical examination.

SYMPTOMS

Cancer of the prostate may produce a wide variety of symptoms. Many of these are the same problems that are caused by urinary blockage or irritation from benign diseases such as BPH or prostatitis. The most common symptoms of prostate disease are a slow urine stream, hesitancy to initiate urination, increased numbers of urinations during day (frequency) or night (nocturia), strong urges to void (urgency), blood in the urine (hematuria), problems with sexual function, and aching pain in the penis, scrotum, testicles, anus, lower abdomen or lower back. The urine stream may be completely shut off ('retention') or there may be a troublesome unintentional dribbling of urine. In addition, advanced cancer may result in fatigue, loss of energy, persistent swelling of one or both lower limbs, and back, rib or hip pain.

It must be emphasized that none of these symptoms are exclusive to cancer and may be caused by benign disorders. It is also important to realize that many men with prostate cancer have no symptoms whatsoever.

SIGNS

Signs are the physical evidence of disease that a physician can detect by examining the patient. Signs of prostate cancer may include a hard growth within the prostate, an enlarged lymph node (*eg* in the neck), a swollen limb,

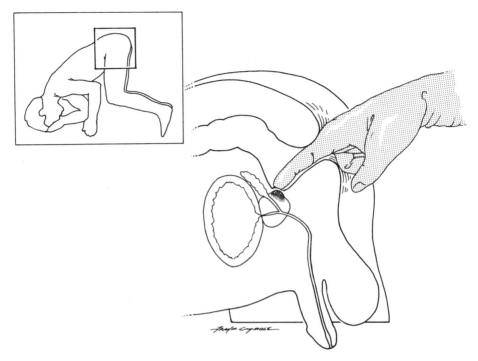

Figure 14. The digital rectal examination.

or a tender spot in the spine, pelvic bone or rib.

The most clear-cut sign of prostate cancer is a **hard lump** in the prostate felt during digital rectal examination. The prostate is easily palpated by placing a gloved, lubricated finger in the rectum and feeling toward the patient's front (fig 14). The examination lasts about 15 seconds and causes an unpleasant, but relatively painless, desire to urinate or defecate. This examination is done with the patient lying on his side, on his back with knees bent, on his stomach with his legs drawn up under the abdomen or standing with legs apart and bent over at the waist. The prostate which ranges from the size of a walnut to the size of a small apple normally has smooth margins and a soft consistency. It is made up of a right and left lobe which are symmetrical (fig 12). A prostate gland with BPH has the consistency of soft rubber and is usually symmetrically enlarged. In contrast, a cancer almost always feels like an asymmetrical area of hard plastic or wood within the gland.

If the cancer has metastasized to the bones, the physician may find a tender area when he presses on the pelvis, spine or ribs. The tenderness indicates an underlying metastasis in the bone. Certainly, if an older man has a persistent pain in a bony spot, a pain that is not necessarily associated with exercise or straining, then he should bring it to the attention of his doctor.

The lymph nodes that are related to the prostate gland lie at the junction of the vessels which drain the tissues of the lower limbs. If prostate cancer plugs these vessels, a backup of fluid, normally drained by the lymphatics, may cause persistent swelling of the legs. There are benign causes of leg swelling, but its presence should prompt a visit to the physician for a full physical examination. When prostate cancer spreads into the **lymphatic vessels** the cancer cells may travel up the lymphatics along the spine, eventually reaching as far as the base of the neck, and they may implant and grow at any point along the way (fig 15).

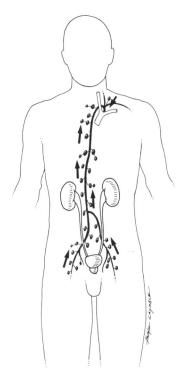

Figure 15. The lymphatic drainage of the prostate gland.

Chapter 12

Diagnostic Studies

When the physician has assessed the patient's symptoms and signs, there may be enough evidence of trouble to warrant a further look in order to confirm or deny the diagnosis of cancer. Initially, the tests that are ordered are intended to investigate urinary symptoms and include: urine tests and blood tests.

URINE TESTS

When a patient provides a sample of his urine for analysis (**urinalysis**) the laboratory checks it for the presence of red or white blood cells which are normal components of blood but should not be found in urine. Finding these cells means that there is either inflammation, or a benign or malignant growth somewhere in the urinary tract (bladder, prostate, or kidneys). Additional tests are required to identify the source of these blood cells. A **urine culture** tests for the presence of bacteria which can cause an infection of the urinary system. The lab 'cultures' the urine at body temperature to allow any bacteria that may be in it to multiply so that they can be easily identified. Normal urine is sterile and nothing should be found growing. If there is bacterial growth during the culture period, a **urinary tract infection** is present. It is not unusual for patients with partially blocked urinary tracts to develop urinary tract infections because they are unable to empty their bladders completely and are thus left with residual urine which can become stagnant and infected.

BLOOD TESTS

Routine blood tests include a **hemoglobin** which measures the oxygen-carrying capacity of red blood cells, a **white blood cell count** which measures the number of infection-fighting white blood cells, and a **platelet count** which shows whether the person has adequate numbers of clotting cells.

Other blood tests include measurements of **electrolytes** to determine the concentration of salts in the blood, and two tests that measure kidney function, the **blood urea nitrogen (BUN)** and **serum creatinine.** BUN and serum creatinine levels will both be higher than normal if the ureters are partially or completely blocked by a prostate growth.

Two blood tests directly address the possible prostate problem by measuring the levels of substances produced by prostatic tissue. These substances normally produced by the cells of the prostate gland are known as **prostatic acid phosphatase (PAP)** and **prostate specific antigen (PSA).** In the presence of benign growths they may be slightly higher than normal, but prostate cancer may lead to high levels of both PAP and PSA in the blood .

PROSTATIC ACID PHOSPHATASE (PAP)

Serum **prostatic acid phosphatase** is an enzyme produced by the prostate gland as well as by other tissues of the body. The original method of detecting PAP involved measurement of its biochemical activity. PAP activity was found to be higher than normal in about 30% of men whose cancer was confined to the prostate, but it was also high in about 25% of elderly men with benign prostate enlargement. Thus, it did not differentiate BPH from prostate cancer in a reliable way.

A second, more accurate means of measuring acid phosphatase was developed in the early 1980s. It involved a technique known as **radioimmunoassay** (RIA) which determined the amount of acid phosphatase present in the serum, rather than its activity. Although this 'RIA-PAP,' or 'the male PAP test' as it has been called, was a significant advance, it was still high in some BPH cases and could not be considered as an accurate means of cancer diagnosis.

Acid phosphatase measurement (by either technique) is useful to patients with advanced disease, because their blood PAP levels may be sufficiently high to be followed. PAP then can serve as an indicator of a positive response to treatment, or the lack of one. It has also been suggested that a high acid phosphatase may be a harbinger of more advanced cancer, even if there is no other evidence of metastases. Thus, if a man is a candidate for surgical treatment but his acid phosphatase is high, then there is more of a chance that his cancer has spread to the lymph nodes. This is a factor that must be taken into account when his treatment is planned.

PROSTATE SPECIFIC ANTIGEN (PSA)

Prostate specific antigen is a protein that is unique to prostatic tissue. The PSA test has recently become the most popular prostate blood test because it is the most specific for cancer and because the test result correlates quite well with the amount of cancer present in the body. It is also a useful guide for treatment since the response to a therapy can be measured as a corresponding decrease of the blood PSA level. Although PSA is specific to the prostate, it is not specific for cancer and it can be high in non-malignant diseases of the prostate. In fact, 20% of men with BPH have a higher than normal level of blood PSA. It is a very sensitive indicator of the number of prostate cells present, benign or malignant. Recent studies showed that 80% of the men who harbor prostate cancer of any stage have correspondingly high blood PSA levels.

If a patient undergoes a radical treatment for localized prostate cancer such as radiation therapy or prostate removal, then the PSA level should fall to normal after treatment, indicating that all the cancer cells were destroyed or removed. If the PSA level does not return to normal, then the physician must search for residual cancer within the prostate, or for cancer cells that were out of reach of the treatment because they had metastasized.

If a patient has metastatic cancer with a high blood level of PSA, then PSA becomes an excellent marker for monitoring treatment response. Almost every patient who responds to appropriate therapy will find that his PSA drops to normal or near-normal levels. Now, by monitoring PSA levels at regular intervals, doctors are able to detect a relapse more quickly than with any other clinical test. It is not unusual for PSA to start rising 6 or 8 months before the patient has any symptoms or signs of recurring cancer. PSA may rise long before PAP.

Physicians usually order tests for blood PSA levels when assessing a patient who has a suspicious nodule on his prostate. A digital rectal examination can lead to a transient rise of blood PSA or PAP levels by forcing these substances out of the gland and into the bloodstream. If cancer is suspected, the physician may wait for two to three days after the physical examination before ordering these tests. The levels will return to normal quite quickly unless there is a continued production by abnormal prostate cells. The laboratory requires several days to process PSA tests so the results will not be available immediately.

Occasionally, a patient with a benign-feeling prostate gland is found to have a high blood PSA level which could indicate a malignancy. The onus is then on the physician to rule out the possibility of a cancer somewhere in the gland. This may require repeated careful rectal examinations by an urologist (prostate and urinary system specialist) and a biopsy (Chapter 13) of any suspicious areas.

Chapter 13

Ultrasound, Cystoscopy, Biopsy

Once the basic urine and blood tests have been done, the physician will proceed with more elaborate methods in an attempt to confirm the diagnosis of cancer. These tests include ultrasound, cystoscopy, and biopsy of the prostate.

TRANSRECTAL ULTRASOUND OF THE PROSTATE

Transrectal ultrasound of the prostate is a relatively new procedure done by an urologist or radiologist trained to analyze the images produced by an ultrasound probe placed into the rectum. This is usually done with the patient lying on his left side or on his back. A well-lubricated probe, about twice the thickness of a finger, is placed through the anus into the rectum (figs 16 & 17). Patients feel a fullness or a desire to void or defecate, but this feeling usually diminishes in a few minutes. The probe contains a crystal which sends out high-frequency sound waves that are either absorbed or reflected back to a receiver in the probe — a principle similar to that of sonar.

The scan gives an image of the prostate gland in cross-section. The gland is scanned along its entire length and width (two planes). If a cancer is present, usually it appears to be less dense (**hypoechoic,** giving less echo) than the surrounding tissues (fig 18a & b). To get a sample for microscopic analysis, the physician can insert a **biopsy needle** alongside the probe and into the suspicious area using direct '**ultrasound guidance**' (fig 19). The patient may feel a sharp, quick jab as the needle passes through the wall of the rectum into the prostate and a small amount of tissue is extracted. Pain is usually transient, gone by the time the procedure is completed. The needle is sufficiently fine and does not damage the rectal wall, and only rarely does it cause rectal bleeding. The patient will often notice some bright red or old brown blood in his urine and semen, or may have transient difficulty urinating for a short time following the biopsy. Many physicians provide patients with antibiotics immediately before, and for one or two doses after the biopsy in order to minimize the chances of an infection, but this rarely occurs.

35

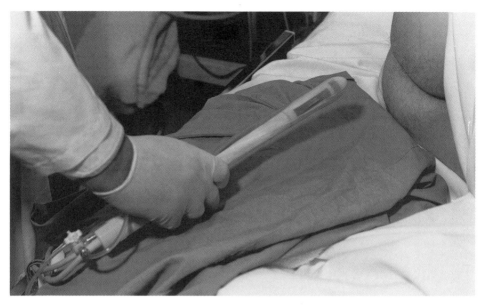

Figure 16. Transrectal ul-
trasound probe.

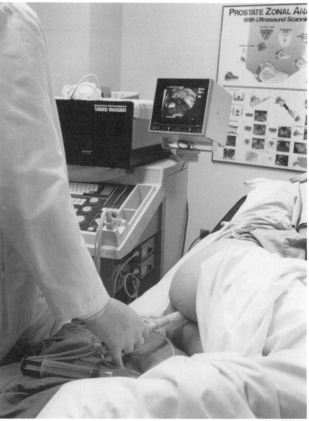

Figure 17. Ultrasound
probe in rectum

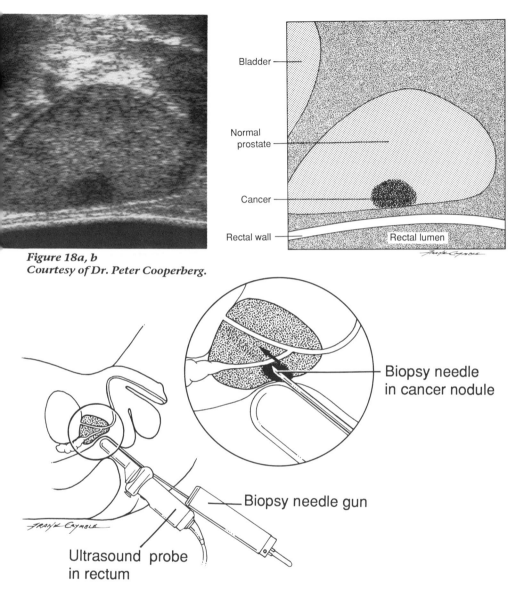

Figure 18a, b
Courtesy of Dr. Peter Cooperberg.

Bladder

Normal prostate

Cancer

Rectal wall

Rectal lumen

Biopsy needle in cancer nodule

Biopsy needle gun

Ultrasound probe in rectum

Figure 19. Ultrasound guided prostate biopsy.

Transrectal ultrasound is *not 100% accurate* and may miss a malignant lesion. If this happens, or if an ultrasound is not done (physician preference or unavailability), the urologist may do a finger-guided biopsy by passing a small needle through the rectum or through the skin just behind the scrotum and into the suspiciously hard area of the gland. As with the ultrasound guided biopsy, the degree of pain is minimal and fleeting, and there is a very low incidence of problems.

Usually, the physician's preference determines whether a biopsy is done with ultrasound or finger guidance. If one biopsy technique fails to detect cancer in a suspicious case, then the other biopsy method should be used. If both procedures are used sequentially, they will confirm a cancer in up to 90% of cases.

When only benign prostatic tissue is found on microscopic analysis of all the biopsies, the patient should be reassessed in 6 months and the biopsy repeated if the suspicious nodule is still present or increasing in size, or if the blood PSA level is increasing.

CYSTOSCOPY

The urologist will also need to visualize the interior of the urinary system. This procedure is called **cystoscopy**. It is usually done in the operating room or in a specially equipped office using a rigid or flexible instrument called a **cystoscope** (fig 20). The cystoscope contains a magnifying lens lit by a light source, and it fits into the urethra through the opening of the penis (fig 21). To better tolerate the procedure, local anesthetic jelly is placed into the urethra and the patient may receive intravenous relaxing medications to help him cope. The procedure takes only 10 to 15 minutes.

Cystoscopy provides the urologist with a great deal of useful information. An assessment can be made of the patency or openness of the urethra, the size of the prostate, and the health of the bladder. These factors may all come into play in the treatment decision process.

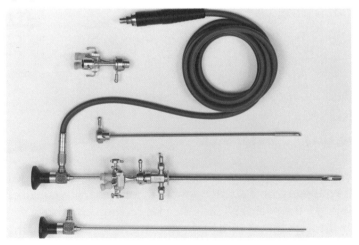

Figure 20. Cystoscope

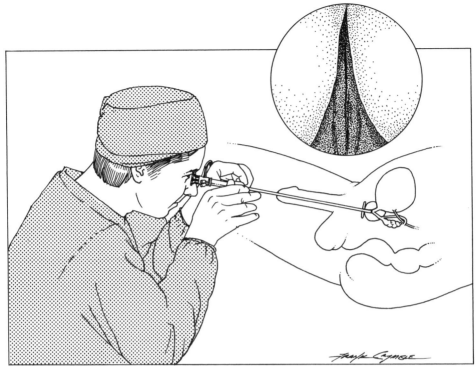

Figure 21. Cystoscope in bladder.

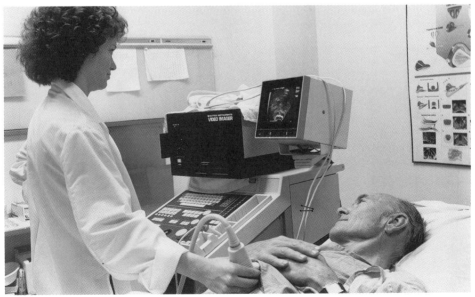

Figure 22. Ultrasound probe on abdomen

39

ABDOMINAL ULTRASOUND

An **abdominal ultrasound** scan is usually done at the same time as the transrectal procedure by passing an ultrasound probe across the abdominal wall (fig 22). This technique can readily generate an image of the kidneys (figs 23A & 23B) and identify any growths, stones or blockages of the ureters (figs 24A & 24B). Furthermore, ultrasound is a sensitive method for detecting liver metastases.

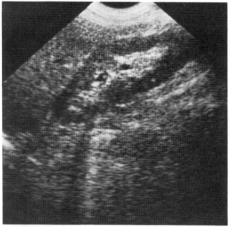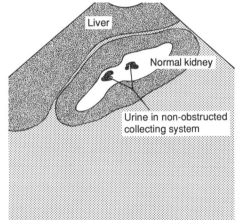

Figure 23 a&b. Normal Kidney ultrasound
Courtesy of Dr. Peter Cooperberg.

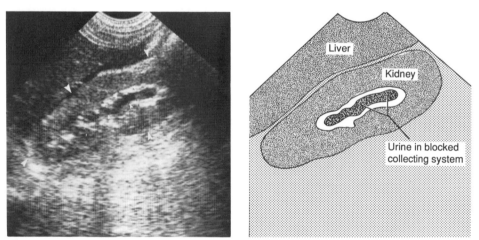

Figure 24a&b. Obstructed Kidney ultrasound
Courtesy of Dr. Peter Cooperberg.

Chapter 14
Staging Tests

Once the prostate cancer is confirmed by biopsy, the physician attempts to take a 'snapshot' of how far it has spread. The amount of cancer that is present within the prostate and the degree of spread are the factors which determine the clinical **stage**. The clinical stage before treatment is based on findings from a combination of digital rectal examination, PSA (and/or PAP) and a **nuclear bone scan**. Additional radiological investigations may include a CT scan, plain x-ray films of the skeleton, and magnetic resonance imaging (MRI). Finally, in some cases the only way to determine the extent of the cancer spread is by exploratory surgery. *The importance of clinical staging cannot be overemphasized* as it has a major influence on both the choice of treatment and the prognosis.

NUCLEAR BONE SCAN

A **nuclear bone scan** is an outpatient procedure done in the hospital's nuclear medicine department. A radioactive material called technetium-99m diphosphonate is injected into an arm vein and the radioactive material sequesters in actively forming bone. Several hours later, the entire skeletal system is scanned painlessly as a slow 'Geiger counter-like' machine called a **gamma camera** passes over the body (fig 25). In prostate cancer, by some unknown mechanism, metastatic cells induce the local bone cells to create new bone (**osteoblastic lesion**) and the result of increased concentration of radioactive material in this area becomes a '**hot spot**' on the scan (figs 26 & 27). Nuclear bone scanning is an extremely sensitive method for detecting cancer that has spread to the bones, but because of its sensitivity it will also detect other bone abnormalities such as arthritis or fractures. Consequently, the cause of a single hot spot on a scan must be investigated further by a plain **x-ray** of the corresponding area. On an x-ray film a prostate cancer metastasis in bone will produce a very dense white lesion compared to arthritis or a fracture. If a bone scan

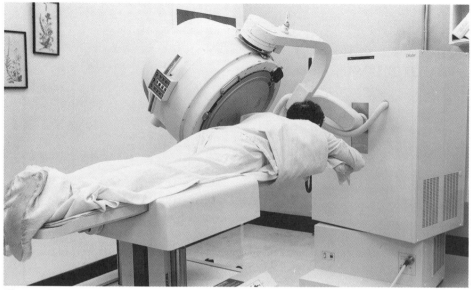

Figure 25. Gamma camera

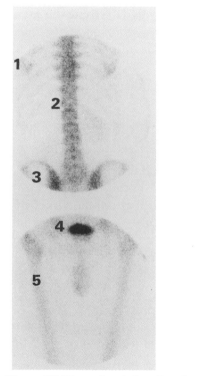

Figure 26. Normal uptake of nuclear material in scapula (1), vertebra (2), ilium (3), bladder (4) and femur (5).

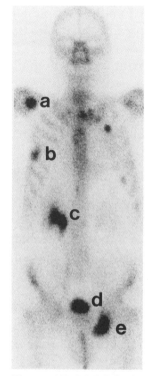

Figure 27. Multiple hot spots on scan (a,b,e). Nuclear material in blocked Kidney (c) and bladder (d).

reveals multiple hot spots, however, the diagnosis of metastatic cancer is almost certain.

Bone scanning is also valuable for the follow-up care of patients undergoing therapy. A physician may arrange for intermittent bone scans over a number of years, or at anytime, should the patient develop pain or other symptoms which suggest bone involvement.

INTRAVENOUS PYELOGRAM

The **intravenous pyelogram (IVP)** is a special x-ray of the urinary system which shows the kidneys, ureters, and bladder, and which is done on an outpatient basis in the radiology department. The procedure lasts approximately one hour and leaves no lingering after-effects. It consists of a series of abdominal x-rays taken after **intravenous contrast** dye is injected into an arm vein. This dye travels through the bloodstream until it is excreted by the kidneys (fig 28a&b). During the period of time that it is being collected and excreted by the kidneys, the dye will reveal an image of the kidneys, ureters

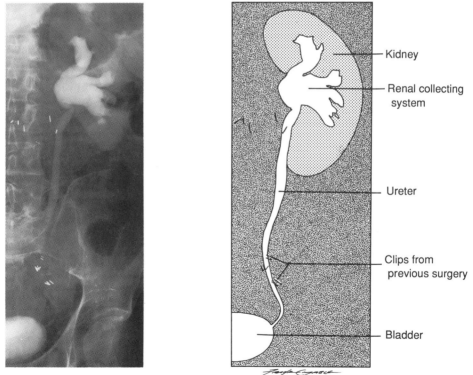

Figure 28a&b. Intravenous pyelogram showing normal left kidney and ureter.

43

and bladder on x-ray. The high-density iodine molecules of the contrast dye appear white on the x-ray film. By providing an image of the anatomy of the kidneys and ureters, the IVP enables the physician to evaluate how well the kidneys are functioning, whether or not there are any blockages due to prostate gland enlargement, and how completely the bladder empties during voiding.

As there are a small number of people who have allergic reactions to the intravenous contrast dye, *any patient who is known to have allergies (to shellfish in particular) should notify his physician* or the radiologist before being injected. If allergies are suspected and the IVP is crucial to the investigation and staging, then the patient can be given special steroid and antihistamine drugs to minimize the chances of an allergic reaction. Although the IVP used to be a standard part of the work-up of prostate cancer, now it is often replaced by an ultrasound examination which is risk-free and may provide all the required information.

COMPUTERIZED AXIAL TOMOGRAPHY ('CAT SCAN,' CT SCAN)

Computerized axial tomography (CAT scan, CT scan) is a sophisticated x-ray procedure that produces cross-sectional images of the human body. It is done in the x-ray department and involves injecting the same contrast material that is used for an IVP. The patient must lie still on the CT table while he very gradually passes through a circular device (fig 29) that takes sequential cross-sectional x-rays (fig 30a&b).

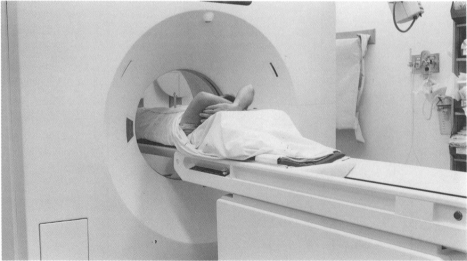

Figure 29. Patient on CT scan gantry.

44

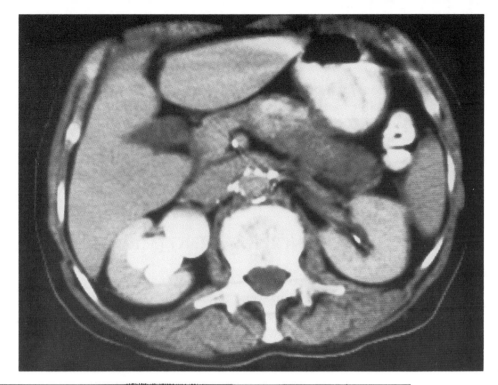

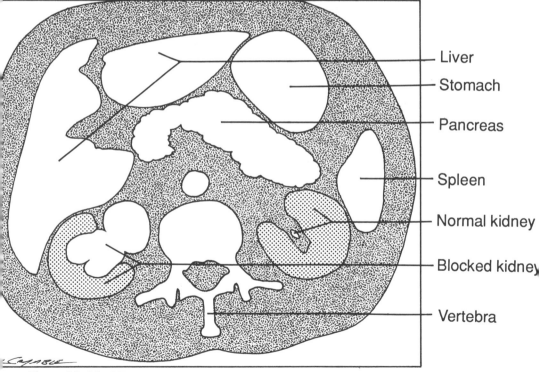

Liver

Stomach

Pancreas

Spleen

Normal kidney

Blocked kidney

Vertebra

Figure 30a&b. CT scan showing normal left kidney and obstructed right kidney.
Courtesy of Dr. Peter Cooperberg.

As a staging tool for prostate cancer, a CT scan may be useful if there is concern about possible metastases that have invaded the lymph nodes in the back of the abdomen ('retroperitoneum') or in pelvis. Small nodes are not necessarily malignant. However, lymph nodes that are markedly enlarged almost always contain metastatic cancer. A CT scan of the pelvis can also provide information about the size of the prostate, the extent of the cancer spread outside of the gland, and the possible involvement of pelvic lymph nodes.

MAGNETIC RESONANCE IMAGING (MRI, MR)

Magnetic resonance imaging (MRI, MR) is a new and very sophisticated test that is being used for staging in some centers. Like CT scanning, it can produce cross sectional body images (or images in any direction!) but with the advantage of delivering absolutely no radiation to the patient. Instead, it works by means of magnetic currents. The patient is positioned in a very powerful electromagnetic field and radio waves are used to detect the responses of the body's protons and electrons to this magnetic field. Different tissues react differently to magnetic fields and thus have different appearances on the scan. In theory, cancerous tissue may respond in a unique way so that its unusual patterns could be distinguished. To date, there is very little experience with MRI in prostate cancer, but there is a lot of work underway. It remains to be seen whether MRI will better CT scan for staging of prostate cancer.

PELVIC LYMPH NODE DISSECTION

If prostate cancer has spread to local lymphatic vessels and lymph nodes, it signifies a higher stage and a worsened prognosis. Such information is extremely important to a physician designing an appropriate treatment protocol for an individual. The probability of lymphatic spread increases with the size of the tumor in the prostate as well as with its pathological grade. For example, a small, one cm, microscopically well-differentiated cancer has less than a 5% chance of having spread to the lymphatics, while a large, poorly-differentiated cancer has an 85% chance of having spread to the lymph nodes by the time the cancer is diagnosed. Large lymph nodes may be detected by a CT scan but in most instances lymph nodes that contain cancer are not large enough to be visualized. The only way to detect and confirm the involvement of these nodes with any certainty is by exploratory surgery. This operation is called a **pelvic lymph node dissection** and may be performed through a standard operative incision or by a new technique known as **laparoscopy**.

A standard pelvic lymph node dissection is done under general or spinal anesthesia. A 5 inch vertical incision is made just above the pubic bone. The area around the prostate is opened up and the lymph nodes on either side against the pelvic sidewall are removed. These lymph nodes are very close to the major blood vessels which lead into and out of the legs as well as to the important **obturator nerve** that controls a portion of the thigh muscles. It is essential that the nodes around the obturator nerves be removed as they are often the only site of spread of the prostate cancer. Great care is taken not to damage the nerve as this would affect the patient's ability to bring his thighs together, making walking difficult. Fortunately, this is an extremely rare complication of the procedure. Other complications, though also rare, can occur and may include wound infections, collection of lymph fluid under the skin or in the pelvis, and swelling of the legs due to blockage of their lymph vessels. After a routine operation and provided there are no complications, the patient remains in hospital for approximately 5 days. Recovery is usually swift and a return to normal activity can be expected in a few weeks.

Laparoscopic surgery has gained tremendous popularity in the last few years. Though the basic technique has been available for some time, it has only recently become popularized because of the development of powerful miniature camera systems, light sources and telescopic lenses. The surgeon performs laparoscopy by making a small incision in the navel, inserting a hollow needle and filling the abdomen with carbon dioxide gas ('pneumoperitoneum'). A small tube with a telescopic lens is then passed through the hole into the abdomen. The attached camera allows the entire abdomen to be viewed on a TV screen. Several secondary holes are made in the abdomen and a variety of snippers, graspers, staplers and suction devices are used to remove the lymph nodes.

In the case of localized cancer, a pelvic lymph node dissection is always done prior to removing the prostate gland. If radiation treatments are recommended, it is important to know whether or not the cancer has spread because this influences the size of the planned radiation field. In some cases, the degree of spread may change the entire course of treatment from one centered on radiating the local prostate tumor to one focusing on treating the entire body by hormone withdrawal or castration (Chapter 26).

Chapter 15
The Stages of Prostate Cancer

Once the urologist has gathered the results of all of the investigations, he can then assign a clinical stage to the patient's cancer (before treatment). The clinical stage reflects the amount of cancer present within the prostate gland itself and how much it has spread to other parts of the body (fig 31). The clinical stage both guides treatment and provides information regarding prognosis.

STAGE A

Stage A is an 'occult' or hidden cancer, that is, *its presence was not suspected during the physical examination*. Instead, it was detected on microscopic examination of prostate tissue removed for some other reason, such as treatment for blockage of the urinary channel by BPH, or with the bladder for bladder cancer (fig 31). If only a few microscopic areas of cancer are found, comprising less than 5% of the entire tissue, and provided that this cancer is 'low-grade' (well-differentiated in its microscopic characteristics), then the cancer is termed a **stage A1** cancer. This is the earliest stage of prostate malignancy that one can have and is unlikely to progress to a higher stage during a patient's lifetime. On the other hand, if more than 5% cancer is found in the tissue specimen, or if the detected cancer is of a higher grade (more poorly-differentiated) it is termed **stage A2**. This disease is more likely to be aggressive and more likely to have an influence on a patient's life span.

STAGE B

A **stage B** cancer is *detected as a hard lump during digital rectal examination of the prostate* (fig 31). If it is confined to one side of the gland, either the left or the right, and it is less than two cm in diameter, then it is considered a **stage B1** cancer. If it involves more than one side of the prostate gland or it is larger than two cm, then it is termed a **stage B2** cancer.

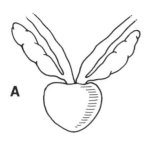

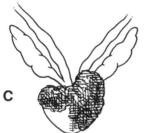

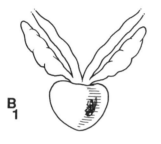

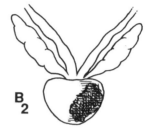

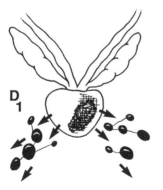

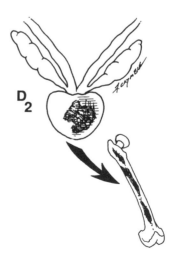

Figure 31. The stages of prostate cancer.

49

Additional Criteria for Stages A and B

The serum PSA and/or prostatic acid phosphatase and bone scan results must be carefully considered in the clinical staging of the cancer. For a cancer to be classified as stage A or B, the PSA measurement must be within normal limits or only minimally elevated. In general terms, the PSA level is proportional to the total amount of cancer present, so a minimal elevation is in keeping with a cancer that is still confined to the prostate. Furthermore, for the cancer to be a stage A or B, the bone scan should show no evidence of hot spots anywhere in the bony skeleton

STAGE C

In **Stage C** the prostate cancer has *grown through the capsule of the gland* and has invaded adjacent structures such as nerves, blood vessels, pelvic muscles, the seminal vesicles or the bladder (fig 31). The tumor may be relatively small but situated peripherally in the gland (**small C**), or it may have replaced large portions of the gland and extensively infiltrated surrounding tissues (**large C**). A patient with a clinical stage C has a normal bone scan and 'limited' increase of the PSA and/or prostatic acid phosphatase level.

STAGE D

In **stage D** prostate cancer there is *metastatic spread of the tumor to other parts of the body,* primarily to the lymph nodes or bones (fig 31). If a CT scan or surgical exploration shows that a patient has positive nodes confined to the pelvis, then his cancer is considered a **stage D1**. If the involved nodes are outside the pelvis, that is, in the back of the abdomen, chest or neck, or if any of his bones are affected, then his cancer is considered to be a **stage D2**.

Chapter 16
Prognosis

Prognosis is a 'forecast' of things to come. It refers to the likelihood of being cured. Physicians 'prognosticate,' or predict the outcome of a disease by assessing the facts of an individual case, and comparing that case to the data accumulated from the study of a multitude of similar cases.

Prostate cancer affects different individuals in different ways. Accordingly, prognostic figures are considered to be generalizations and must be considered in light of the general health of the individual, the stage of the cancer and the form of therapy. Survival figures are usually presented in terms of the chances of surviving 5, 10 or 15 years after the diagnosis is established and the treatment instituted. One must always remember that prostate cancer tends to strike the elderly who may already have a high incidence of death-causing conditions such as heart disease.

IMPORTANT CONSIDERATIONS WHEN INTERPRETING SURVIVAL FIGURES

Survival tables are based on the disease progress of many individuals, not just one or two. The large numbers are necessary to be able to provide an average performance among a group of people who have many differences. The tables are useful to predict what can be expected for 100 cancer patients with a specific stage. Thus, a 5-year survival rate of 60% means that of 100 patients with that particular stage of cancer, 60 would be expected to survive 5 years. They are not designed to predict how an *individual* patient will do. Any particular individual could be one of the 60 survivors or one of the 40 who do not survive. As well, in any group of cancer patients, there will always be the 'outriders,' those individuals who, by virtue of some unquantified characteristics, respond differently from the rest.

Many physicians have had patients with tiny, early-stage cancers who died of a recurrence;, while others who were expected to die of cancer 'beat the odds' and outlived even their surgeons.

51

In the final analysis, no one can tell any individual patient who has a potentially curable prostate cancer, how he will fare. Physicians can only quote the odds. With the current state of knowledge, only time can tell what the outcome will be for any single patient.

THE SURVIVAL FIGURES

The 10-year survival rate for patients with microscopic, well-differentiated cancer limited to the prostate and with no evidence of metastases (stage A1) is 90%. In other words, men with stage A1 tumors may have close to normal life expectancy. Cancer death within 10 years of a radical prostatectomy, however, may occur in 15% of stage A2 cases. When the tumor is of small volume, and is contained within the gland, and when there are no lymph nodes involved and no other metastases (stage B1), the 10-year survival rate is roughly 80% after radical therapy. If a man has a stage B2 cancer, his chances of surviving 10 years drop to 60%. Spread of cancer through the capsule of the gland but without metastases (stage C) gives a 10-year survival of between 35% and 45%. When lymph nodes are involved (stage D1), the 10-year figures are 20% to 30%. Finally, when there are metastases in the bones or other organs (stage D2), the 5 and 10-year survival statistics are 20% and 5% respectively.

WHAT ABOUT THE INCURABLE CANCER?

It has to be admitted that at our present state of knowledge, some cases of prostate cancer are simply not curable. These are the cases in which there are numerous metastases. It is only fair for a physician to respond truthfully to a patient when there is considerable certainty that his cancer cannot be cured. For the incurable cases, the treatment is palliative and aimed at improving the quality of life rather than at curing the cancer.

How long can a person live with incurable prostate cancer? The commonly asked question, "How long do I have to live?" is one that most physicians are reluctant to answer because their predictions have been proven wrong so many times. However, for patients who need to make realistic plans for their own and their family's future, some indication of life-expectancy is important. It is fairly safe to assume that almost no one with incurable disease will live for more than 10 years. Two years is what can be expected by at least half of all the incurable patients; with very few surviving more than 7 or 8 years.

Chapter 17
Detecting a Silent Enemy - Screening

WHAT IS SCREENING?

By the time symptoms appear, cancer can be well-established and, in many cases, may have already spread to other parts of the body. In order to increase the chances of cure, prostate cancer must be identified in its earliest phases, *before* symptoms occur. **Screening** is looking for cancer in asymptomatic (symptom-free) individuals.

Abundant evidence supports the concept of screening. First, prostate cancer is of sufficient magnitude to warrant the dedication of public health resources for screening. In 1991 alone, more than 106,000 new cases and over 30,000 deaths were attributed to this disease in the United States and 11,300 and 3,600, respectively in Canada. The US National Cancer Institute has estimated that the risk of a newborn child developing clinically detected cancer of the prostate some time during his life is 9%. Second, the disease often exists in a long, symptom-free phase during which it can be easily detected and cured. Unlike most other parts of the body in which cancer can develop, there is ready access to the prostate if one cares to examine it. Finally, a simple blood test for a marker of prostate cancer activity (PSA) is also now available.

For several years urologists have been interested in the development of some method of screening the entire male population in order to detect prostate cancer at an early stage. Unfortunately, from both a practical and economic point of view, this screening process is very difficult to apply to large populations of men. First, the benefits of detecting cancer at an early stage must be balanced against the costs and risks of diagnosis and treatment. It would be very expensive to give each and every man a physical examination, blood tests, ultrasound and x-rays, and patients who undergo a biopsy face some risk of complications.

Second, prostate cancer represents a heterogeneous disease whose behavior is difficult to predict. If we were to find every non-symptomatic prostate cancer that is present in the male population, we would be including many cancers that are small and so slow-growing that the affected individual would die of something else without ever knowing that he had it! At the other extreme, of all the men that are currently found to have prostate cancer, half already have cancer that is too extensive to be cured. Screening would be of no benefit to these individuals.

Our ideal goals in screening would be to detect cancers before they are too advanced for cure, while at the same time to *not* detect a "tiny" cancer that is not destined to become dangerous during a man's lifetime. Current evidence indicates that a cancer that is at least one cubic centimeter in volume is likely to grow and develop into a significant disease over a period of 10 to 15 years.

INHERENT PROBLEMS WITH SCREENING

There are a number of biases built into screening programs. The first is **lead time bias** the artificial increase of *apparent* survival time which is due to earlier-than-usual detection of the disease rather than a real prolongation of life. The second problem is **length bias**: screening programs are more likely to identify indolent diseases, thereby over-representing the cases that have the least aggressive cancers and therefore the longest survival. Finally, there is **patient selection bias**: the screened population is not necessarily representative of the general population. Apparently, people who submit to screening are more informed or more health-conscious than people who do not. Thus, any apparent benefit from screening may be due, in part, to the characteristics of the individuals *being* screened, rather than due to the screening program itself.

As a result of these inherent problems, critics charge that it has never been satisfactorily shown that screening for cancer saves or prolongs life. These detractors suggest that there is not sufficient justification for putting patients through the expense, inconvenience, embarrassment, pain and potential risk of various screening tests.

Despite these criticisms, the medical community is acutely aware of the fact that during the past 50 years no treatment has been able to significantly alter the death rate of advanced prostate cancer. Until the 'silver bullet' that will eradicate this disease is found, the only hope of improving survival lies in identifying cancers early, before there has been spread. For this reason, screening is pursued, hoping that the right test and the right program will make a difference.

WHAT MAKES GOOD SCREENING TESTS?

The value of a screening test lies in its ability to differentiate people who have the particular disease from people who do not. The parameters used to evaluate the effectiveness of a screening test are sensitivity and specificity.

Sensitivity refers to the proportion of individuals with the disease who have a *positive* test result - the likelihood of identifying people who have the disease.

Specificity refers to the proportion of individuals without the disease who have a *negative* result. In other words, it is the test's ability to show that healthy people are healthy.

The ideal screening test must be sensitive enough to detect almost all the cancers that are present in the studied population. It must also be highly specific, minimizing the number of falsely positive tests that result in unnecessary biopsies. A test that is highly sensitive but not specific enough will single out too many healthy people, subjecting them to needless and possibly harmful diagnostic work-ups. Thus, when screening thousands of people, it is preferable for specificity to be high, even at the cost of some sensitivity.

In addition to the ability to identify disease, screening tests must be well-tolerated and safe. When the chances of his having the disease are small, no asymptomatic individual in his right mind would submit to a screening test that is painful or dangerous. Moreover, unless the test is quick and simple, no one will bother to show up. Finally, as hundreds or thousands of tests are done in a screening program, the test must be inexpensive.

THE SCREENING TESTS

Digital Rectal Examination

Digital rectal examination has been studied as a screening tool. Though it may be quite specific for prostate cancer, it is not sensitive enough to detect all cases since only a minority of cases are palpable. Nevertheless, it is readily available and it does not require an unreasonable effort for men over 40 to have an annual physical examination including a rectal examination.

Blood Tests

Blood tests for tumor markers produced by the prostate, such as **acid phosphatase** and **prostate specific antigen**, have also been considered for screening. Acid phosphatase has been judged not specific enough to be used widely as a screening tool. Prostate specific antigen, however, is more likely to make a significant impact on the early detection of prostate cancer, particularly when combined with a rectal examination. Fortuitously, this combination of tests will not detect all prostate cancers, but most likely just those that are larger than one cubic centimetre and thus destined to become significant within 10 to 15 years.

Transrectal Ultrasound

A third suggested method for screening groups of patients has been **transrectal ultrasound** examination of the prostate. Unfortunately transrectal ultrasound also lacks sufficient specificity because it finds many 'suspicious' areas in benign prostate glands. If transrectal ultrasound were widely used to look for early cancers, too many men would undergo unnecessary biopsies. In addition the financial *cost of screening* men aged 50 to 70 with transrectal ultrasound plus the cost of subsequent treatment is estimated to be in the billions of dollars.

IPG RECOMMENDATIONS FOR PROSTATE SCREENING

Ongoing studies are looking at the role of screening in prostate cancer. Researchers hope that they will answer the question of whether earlier detection can truly improve prostate cancer mortality rates but the answer may not be available for another 10 years. What we know now is that prostate cancer is generally slow-growing and many patients will die with it rather than from it. Available data suggests that a cancer that has grown to a size of 1 cubic centimetre in volume will probably have a deleterious impact on an individual's life within 10 to 15 years. It is therefore recommended, based on the best currently available information, that men between the ages of 50 and 70 should have an annual prostate specific antigen (PSA) blood test and a digital rectal examination of the prostate done by a competent physician.

SECTION V:
TREATMENT OVERVIEW

Chapter 18
General Treatment Overview

It is important to realize that there is more than one way to treat prostate cancer. Choosing the optimum **therapy** requires consideration of many factors including the man's age, current and past general health, the stage and grade of the cancer, and the social and emotional needs of the patient and his family. Furthermore, the recommendations of his physician or local cancer clinic will be influenced by their own treatment experience and biases.

Thus, if a man speaks to different physicians or he reads different manuals or listens to his friends, he may be surprised (and very confused) by the variety of choices available to him. His own personal situation and desires are important. Some men opt for a very conservative approach. Others choose to undergo the most aggressive therapy available.

Fortunately, prostate cancer is one of the more responsive cancers. In its early stages it can be cured with aggressive therapy and in its later stages it can be well-controlled for extended periods of time. Once the cancer is diagnosed, the investigations may take some time to complete. There is generally no need to rush into any particular treatment. A thoughtful, considered approach should be taken, keeping in mind that the cancer has likely existed for months or years before diagnosis and things are not going to change during the relatively short time required to make informed decisions about treatment.

Treatment options include surgery, radiation therapy, hormone-withdrawal therapy, chemotherapy and expectant observation. Sometimes a combination of treatments is used.

SURGERY

Surgical therapy (Chapter 21) may involve a **transurethral operation** in which a core of tissue is removed from the prostate (through the urethra, the urine channel of the penis) to permit normal urination. **Exploratory surgery** may be done through an incision in the lower abdominal wall to remove the lymph nodes for staging purposes. The same lymph nodes may be examined through a small hole in the abdomen using a tiny telescopic lens and camera system known as a **laparoscope**. If the cancer is confined to the prostate, the surgeon may do a '**radical prostatectomy**,' removing the entire prostate and seminal vesicles. In special circumstances, if radiation has been tried but has failed to control the disease, the prostate can be removed using a procedure known as '**salvage prostatectomy**.' For advanced, metastatic cancer, surgical removal of the testicles may be appropriate.

RADIATION THERAPY

In certain cases **radiation therapy** is used with a curative intent. Patients with localized cancer who may not be strong enough to withstand surgery or men who have too much disease to be surgically curable or who are anxious to avoid surgery, are all candidates for radiation therapy (Chapter 25). Also, in patients who have undergone surgical excision of the prostate, radiation may be added to their treatment if it is discovered that the cancer has not been entirely removed.

In cases of metastatic cancer, radiation may be used to shrink metastatic deposits that are causing symptoms such as pain or blockage of an organ system. This use of radiation is **palliative** rather than curative. It is designed to keep a patient comfortable and to improve his quality of life rather than to lengthen his life or to provide a cure.

HORMONE-WITHDRAWAL THERAPY

Hormone-withdrawal therapy (Chapter 26) usually involves **castration** (removal of the testicles). In most cases of advanced cancer, this produces a prolonged **remission** (the disease seems to disappear or to hold still for a time). Reversible forms of castration by means of drugs are being investigated for both early and advanced stages of cancer.

CHEMOTHERAPY

Chemotherapy is not a common means of treating prostate cancer (Chapter

27). Chemotherapy drugs may be offered to men who suffer relapses and increasing symptoms after having been treated by hormone-withdrawal therapy. These drugs are synthetic and differ both in terms of chemistry and effect from hormones. Unfortunately, no **chemotherapeutic agent** (chemotherapy drug) has yet shown great promise in the management of prostate cancer, but there are some cases where they may be considered.

EXPECTANT OBSERVATION

A man and his doctor must always consider the option of no treatment, or delayed treatment. The **no treatment option** is particularly prudent for the very old man who is suffering from other debilitating diseases. In such a situation it is most likely that the patient will die from causes other than prostate cancer.

Chapter 19
Stage-Specific Treatment

STAGE A

Stage A represents an 'occult' or hidden prostate cancer, whose presence was not suspected during the regular examination. By chance, the cancer is detected during microscopic examination of a prostate tissue sample removed as part of the treatment for blockage of the urinary channel (Chapter 21; fig 31). Since the diagnosis of cancer was not entertained before the surgery, the diagnosis comes as a shock to the patient (and sometimes to the doctor).

Stage A1

If less than 5% of the sample is cancerous and if the cancer cells are well-differentiated, then this is stage A1. The treatment at stage A1 depends on the age of the patient, his general medical condition and his desire for future sexual activity. It is estimated that stage A1 disease will progress to a higher stage or even metastasize in 15% of cases. However, it might take 10 to 15 years to do so. For this reason, if an elderly man is diagnosed as having stage A1 prostate cancer, it is reasonable for his doctor to treat him no further, and simply to observe him, examining the prostate and evaluating the tumor markers (*eg* PSA) annually. The physician may need to intervene if signs of advancing local or metastatic disease develop at a later date.

For a younger individual who would have a life expectancy of more than 10 to 15 years, a case can be made for more radical intervention including radical prostatectomy or radiation therapy. For younger patients, some urologists advocate doing a repeat transurethral resection (TUR) or ultrasound-guided biopsies of the prostate before going on to more aggressive therapy. This gives the urologist a second look for residual cancer cells that would change the stage of the disease to A2 and thus would justify more aggressive treatment. If no further cancer is found after repeat biopsy or resection, then the doctor may have greater confidence electing to just observe this patient. It should be noted, however, that even if there is no residual cancer on a repeat transurethral prostatectomy, approximately 20% of patients will have undetected cancer cells in the prostate tissue that remains behind. On the other hand, of patients who do have some tumor found on a repeat resection and do undergo a radical prostatectomy, approximately 5% have no residual cancer in the removed prostate gland! Both these scenarios represent extremes and it is generally recommended that a younger man with stage A1 prostate cancer, with or without a repeat staging TUR, be considered for a radical prostatectomy. The alternatives are radical radiation therapy, or observation with intervention when there is evidence that the disease is advancing.

The treatment of stage A1 disease remains a controversial topic and one worthy of extensive discussions with one's physicians before making a final decision. It is important to remember that at this stage, the disease is in the early, slow growing phase of its natural history so that one has several months during which to make a carefully considered decision. Seeking a **second opinion** from a respected authority may be useful in helping to come to a final decision regarding treatment.

Stage A2

If more than 5% of the prostate specimen removed by prostatectomy shows cancer, or if the pathology shows cancer cells that are poorly-differentiated, then the cancer is at stage A2. At least 35% of patients with this stage will eventually progress to more extensive cancer, including metastatic disease. For this reason, intervention should be aggressive unless the patient is unfit or refuses such treatment. Suggested treatment is either a radical prostatectomy or some form of radiation therapy directed at the prostate. A less commonly used, but still worthwhile alternative is surgical or medical hormone-withdrawal therapy (castration). This latter option is particularly practical for an older man who is no longer sexually active and may not be fit enough to undergo radical surgery or radiation therapy.

Surgical Exploration

Soon after the diagnosis is made, in both stages A1 and A2 it is important to assess the serum prostate specific antigen (PSA) and/or acid phosphatase levels. If these markers are above normal, then the disease is probably more extensive than might be clinically apparent. Surgical exploration of the pelvic lymph nodes by an open incision or by laparoscopy should be considered unless the bone scan or CT scan show evidence of cancer spread to bones or lymph nodes, making more exploration superfluous. Surgical exploration of the pelvic nodes can be done in conjunction with a radical prostatectomy or prior to radiation therapy. If the nodes are cancerous then the disease is reclassified to stage D1 and appropriate treatment is started.

STAGE B

A **stage B** tumor is a hard lump detected by digital rectal examination of the prostate (figs 14 & 31). The lump is sometimes called a "nodule". If it is confined to one side of the gland and if it is less than two cm in diameter, then it is considered to be a **stage B1** nodule. If it is confined by the outer limits of the gland but appears to involve more than one side of the prostate or if it is larger than 2 cm, then it is termed a **stage B2** nodule.

Like stage A prostate cancer, stage B cancer is potentially curable if it is treated by either radical prostatectomy or radiation therapy. For **stage B1** disease, a radical prostatectomy will render the patient disease-free in upwards of 75% of cases. Presumably, the other 25% have metastases already present at the time of the surgery but in amounts too small to be detected by physical examination, blood tests, nuclear bone scan or x-ray. With time, these cells will grow and develop into tumors which may be in the pelvic lymph nodes, other lymph nodes or bones.

In clinical **stage B2** the chances of a man being totally free of disease 15 years after treatment is only 25%. Nevertheless, many of these patients will continue to thrive even with small amounts of progressive or metastatic cancer within their bodies and will have been provided many good years by the initial aggressive therapy.

The more cancer there is in the prostate, or the more poorly-differentiated the cells appear under the microscope, the more likely it is that the cancer is already spread at the time of diagnosis. An alternative to radical prostatectomy or radical radiation therapy for such patients is hormone-withdrawal treatment. For the older, less physically fit person, or someone with a limited life-expectancy because of other significant illness, observation alone may be considered an appropriate option in treating stage B prostate cancer.

STAGE C

In Stage C, the prostate cancer has grown through the capsule of the gland and invades adjacent structures such as nerve fibres, blood vessels, pelvic muscle, the seminal vesicles or the bladder (fig 31). The tumor may be relatively small and peripherally placed in the gland (**small C**), or it may replace large portions of the gland and extensively infiltrate the surrounding tissues (**large C**). In stage C, the bone scan is normal and there is limited rise of the PSA and/or acid phosphatase level.

It is generally accepted that stage C prostate cancer cannot be totally eliminated by radical prostatectomy or radiation therapy. However, if there is no evidence of metastases to lymph nodes, bone, or other sites, then there is an excellent outlook for long-term control of the disease.

If tests fail to reveal cancer spread beyond the prostate, there are three treatment options: 1) Observation alone, especially for the very elderly patient who is unfit, and who has no urinary symptoms. If, however, the patient does have symptoms then some form of therapy will have to be given. 2) Radiation therapy by external beam may be administered: it is the preferred method of treatment. In selected cases, radiation may be given by interstitial implants (Chapter 25). 3) Hormone withdrawal may be considered for the man who does not want, or may not tolerate radiation therapy.

Radiation therapy is a particularly good choice if the cancer is well-differentiated and PSA and PAP are normal or minimally elevated. Such patients do well with radiation directed only at the prostate, as it is statistically unlikely that the tumor has spread to the lymph nodes. For the patient who has a poorly-differentiated cancer and/or very high tumor markers however, there is a high probability that the disease has already spread to his lymph nodes and possibly to his bones. In this circumstance, the physician may use radiation therapy to the prostate gland to control a tumor that is blocking the urethra and may at the same time institute hormone-withdrawal therapy to deal with the probable cancer spread. In some cancer treatment centers radiation therapy would be directed at both the prostate and the surrounding pelvic tissue to try to shrink any cancerous lymph nodes, reserving hormone-withdrawal therapy for when, and if, metastatic disease is identified. In other centers, hormone-withdrawal therapy would be started 'up front,' withholding radiation treatments for later palliation.

Finally, a middle-of-the-road situation exists when the cancer is moderately well-differentiated and/or the serum tumor markers are only moderately elevated. In this situation the odds are approximately 50:50 that the cancer has spread to the lymph nodes. In this case it would be worthwhile for the surgeon to do a lymph node dissection in order to know, with more certainty, whether or not the cancer has spread. This is important from a psychological point of view as well as from a treatment planning and prognostic point of view. If the cancer has spread, then it might be advisable to go directly to hormone-withdrawal therapy, reserving any form of radiation for a later day when it could be needed to control the disease at the prostate level.

If the lymph nodes are negative, however, then the best course would be to proceed to radical radiation therapy with the hope of curing the cancer or holding it in check for many years.

STAGE D

In **stage D** prostate cancer there is metastatic tumor spread to other parts of the body, primarily to the lymph nodes in the pelvis, other lymph nodes of the body, and the bony skeleton (fig 31). Once prostate cancer has spread beyond the prostate, a cure is unlikely. In this situation, all treatment approaches are considered to be palliative, designed to control the symptoms and to maximize the quality of life rather than to provide a cure. Since the disease has spread beyond the prostate gland, it is impossible to completely remove all of the cancer by surgery.

Stage D1

In **stage D1** the cancer has spread to the lymph nodes within the pelvis but to no other parts of the body. In this stage, if sexual function is not of primary concern to the patient, initiation of hormone-withdrawal therapy should be used to delay the development of further metastases and symptoms of the disease. There are advocates of administering radiation therapy which is directed at the whole pelvis with an extra boost to the prostate for stage D1 cancer. This is intended to treat as many of the lymph nodes as possible and to hopefully prevent the cancer from spreading further.

Stage D2

When the tumor has spread to other parts of the body, usually to the bone, the cancer is a clinical **stage D2** (fig 31). It is not uncommon for patients in this situation to be weak, tired, and to have bone pain, loss of appetite and weight, and difficulty urinating. The most common treatment for stage D2 is hormone-withdrawal therapy. While it cannot cure the cancer, it can slow cellular growth and reduce the size of many of the cancer sites. It also helps to extend life and to improve the quality of life by relieving the symptoms.

Hormone Therapy

The most effective way to reduce testosterone is to surgically remove the testicles (castration). Alternatively, medications may be taken, although these may produce side-effects (Chapter 26). Regardless of the means by which testosterone is reduced, loss of sexual desire, impotence, and hot flushes often result. Hormone-withdrawal therapy will lead to a dramatic response in 85% of cases. Patients with severe bone pain will have relief within days or weeks, relief which can last anywhere from 6 months to 10 years, although the average is 24 months. Eventually the cancer adapts to its new hormone-reduced environment and begins to grow again in response to the very small amounts of testosterone still in the blood or even without any serum testosterone at all.

When someone who has been treated by hormone withdrawal shows signs of disease progression, an alternative form of anti-hormone treatment may be instituted with the rationale that further testosterone reduction may kill some of the developing cancer cells. Of patients who develop progressive disease after their testicles have been removed, 20% respond for a short time to an antiandrogen drug. Conversely, in a similar percentage of cases, patients treated initially by a medical form of castration, such as estrogens or antiandrogens, may respond to surgical removal of the testicles, or treatment with a LHRH agonist. Unfortunately, the addition of a third form of hormone deprivation treatment is almost never successful.

Chemotherapy

Only 15% of men with prostate cancer respond well to chemotherapy. On the average, the response lasts only 6 months. Some of the chemotherapeutic drugs that are being used in a variety of centers around the world include adriamycin, cyclophosphamide, 5-fluorouracil, mitoxantrone and mitomycin C. There are substantial side-effects to these drugs, particularly for the elderly, and they must be used with caution. Sometimes they are useful to younger men who are suffering from relapsing prostate cancer which is resistant to hormone treatments. They should be medically fit and should discuss the potential side-effects of chemotherapy with the physician.

New Approaches

There are a number of novel treatment approaches on the horizon for the treatment of stage D prostate cancer. Scientists have been studying a variety of 'growth factors' that stimulate the growth of cancer cells and may be important to cancers which are no longer sensitive to testosterone (Chapter 29).

An antiparasitic used since the first half of this century, called Suramin™, is undergoing clinical study. It was found to inhibit several types of growth factors but unfortunately, preliminary trials in patients have been unimpressive. The addition of a material known as 'TNF' (tumour necrosis factor) to Suramin™ therapy may enhance its effects. Research continues into the development of related compounds with more specific anti-cancer properties.

Another novel approach being studied involves attaching a chemotherapeutic drug to an antibody which, for instance, binds to prostate specific antigen. In this way, at least theoretically, the antibody will stick only to prostate cancer cells, which the attached drug will destroy (Chapter 27).

Stimulation of the immune system is also being tried for a variety of different cancers because the ability of the body's immune system to fight disease may be compromised in cancer patients. It is hoped that one day there may be a role for immunotherapy in the management of advanced prostate cancer but, to date, this remains in the investigative stage.

SECTION VI: SURGERY

Chapter 20

Preparation for Surgery

ADMISSION TO HOSPITAL

In some hospitals, admission for surgery can be booked ahead of time by the surgeon's staff. The patient will be given a date and time to present himself at the admissions desk of the hospital. In other hospitals, patients are placed on a waiting list for surgery and are contacted by phone to come into hospital when a bed becomes available.

The waiting list system may only give short notice of when a bed is free, therefore it is important for the patient to remain within reach so that the hospital can contact him promptly. He should keep his schedule flexible pending the admission. It is not uncommon for a call to be put out as late as the morning before the next day's surgery. The admissions clerk will request that the patient report to the hospital that very afternoon to be prepared for surgery.

Welcome to chaos?

A variety of admission procedures are required of new arrivals, so come prepared with all the patience you can muster. People will ask you questions, lots of questions. Some you will have already answered many times over. There may be delays, foul-ups, snarky personnel and people who seem totally unconcerned with the seriousness of your problem. Most disturbing of all, is that growing feeling in your gut that everyone working in the place is totally incompetent. What to do when this happens? Take hold of yourself. Relax. Welcome to THE HOSPITAL!

Hospitals are big places with lots of things going on. Particularly in major centers where emergencies are frequent, the priorities of physicians, nurses, orderlies and admitting clerks may be suddenly altered, leaving you in a frustrating holding pattern. If you conclude that the place is complete chaos, you will not be the first to have done so.

The best way to get through the preoperative period in hospital (and much of the stay after surgery) is to just grin and bear it. Your lifeline is your confidence in your surgeon and the knowledge that *somehow* the environment is geared to providing the right treatment at the right time. While you may be sitting in the lurch wondering why you have been deserted suddenly, there may be some poor soul down the hall who requires the immediate attention of the 15 highly-qualified people at his bedside. This is what hospitals are all about. The force and energy of critical services and personnel will be mustered for you when you need it (but often not before).

You will learn a lot about life if you become a careful observer of hospital activity. Watch your fellow patients carefully and you may be counting your blessings before you know it. During the course of your stay you will probably also come across a few examples of some of the outstanding individuals who have adapted to and flourish in this unique environment.

Hospital Admission

Your first meeting will be with the admissions clerk. Identification and basic personal information is recorded. Financial or insurance information may be requested. You will then be directed to or escorted to your hospital room.

Nursing Admission

Once you are on the ward, a nurse carries out a nursing admission. She (or he) records basic information regarding your health and current problem. She then performs a brief examination that includes a measurement of your weight and assessment of your 'vital signs' (heart rate, breathing rate, blood pressure and temperature).

Doctor Admission

In a non-university hospital, a copy of the surgeon's office consultation note will have been sent to the hospital and this will serve as the source of medical information about your problem and any physical examinations that you may have had. The surgeon may be required to update that information after you arrive.

In a university hospital, a medical admission is done by either the medical student, intern or surgical resident (trainee). You will be asked to relate your symptoms again. A list of the tests already done will be recorded along with the responses to a variety of basic medical questions. Then the examiner will do a physical examination. Depending on the organization of the particular teaching program at the hospital, the residents may come around later as a group to see you, often with the chief urology resident. The chief resident is in his last year of surgery training and is responsible for assuring that an appropriate medical admission and interpretation of questions and findings is made, along with organizing last minute tests and preparations for surgery.

PREPARATION FOR SURGERY

Blood Cross-match

In most cases, blood will be 'cross-matched' for your surgery. This means that a sample of your blood will be tested and compatible blood found and reserved for you in case a blood transfusion is required during or after your operation.

In the old days surgeons used to 'top up' patients who had a slightly low blood count before or after surgery. Today, as a result of the small but real hazards associated with blood transfusions (see **HIGHLIGHT How Safe is a Blood Transfusion?**), along with the expense and difficulty of obtaining blood, physicians and surgeons have modified their use of blood and blood products significantly and now give blood only when it is absolutely necessary. Instead they have come to rely increasingly on the patient's natural ability to restore his own blood level, even though this takes more time.

As a result of the AIDS crisis, programs have been developed in which patients can 'bank' their own blood before an operation so that if blood is required, they receive their own blood back. The timing for this sort of thing can be tricky for cancer patients since enough time between the donation and surgery must pass to allow the patients to build up their blood level again for operation. Since cancer surgery is usually carried out within a few weeks of diagnosis, there may not be enough time. To find out whether there is a personal blood banking system in your area and whether you are a suitable candidate, speak to your surgeon and the local Red Cross or hospital blood bank.

You have the right to refuse blood if you wish. If that is your choice, you should ensure that your surgeon and other medical personnel are clearly notified of this. In order to legally protect the doctor and hospital, you may be required to sign a disclaimer to this effect.

How Safe is a Blood Transfusion?

Dana V. Devine Ph.D.

Sometime during the course of treatment for cancer you may require blood transfusions. Blood for transfusion is collected from volunteer donors at a transfusion center or at the Red Cross and separated into three components: red blood cells, platelets and plasma. Red blood cells contain hemoglobin, the red, oxygen-carrying protein. Transfusion of red cells is used to correct anemia caused either by blood loss or by inadequate blood cell production. Platelets help blood to clot. Plasma is the fluid part of the blood: it is yellow and contains clotting proteins, antibodies and other important substances. When a patient receives a transfusion, the hospital blood bank checks the donated blood for compatibility with the patient's blood.

Many people have questions concerning the safety of blood used in transfusions. All blood that is transfused in North America comes from volunteer donors. This practice was instituted to reduce the risk of transfusion-related hepatitis which is higher when donors are paid. In addition, all volunteer blood donors are screened before giving blood: a lifestyle that places the potential donor at risk of contracting transmissible diseases eliminates that individual from donating blood. There are some special cases when people receive payment for plasma donations. However, their plasma is not transfused, it is used for the production of isolated blood proteins.

All blood collected is tested for transmissible diseases such as syphilis, hepatitis B, hepatitis C (formerly called 'non-A, non-B hepatitis'), human immunodeficiency virus (the AIDS virus), and human T-cell leukemia virus (HTLV-1). Because the tests used for these diseases are very sensitive, the chances of contracting any of them from tested blood is very, very small. For instance, the estimated risk of contracting AIDS from a blood transfusion is less than 1 in 1,000,000. In the recent past, the most common illness that arose following a transfusion was 'transfusion-related hepatitis' (non-A, non-B hepatitis). In the late 1980s, the virus that causes this was discovered and named hepatitis C virus and now all blood is routinely screened for it. Some blood is also tested for cytomegalovirus (CMV). CMV infection is like a cold, but the virus can remain dormant in blood cells. While most people are naturally infected with CMV before old age, it is important to test blood for the presence of this virus because it can be dangerous to people who have a compromised immune system (the AIDS patient).

The discovery that AIDS can be transmitted in blood changed the practice of blood transfusion. Some unfortunate people contracted AIDS from transfusions before anyone knew that AIDS was caused by a blood-borne virus, and before there was a test for HIV. Now, there has been a leveling-off or an actual decline in the amount of red blood cells transfused in North America. Physicians and surgeons have become reluctant to give blood unless it is truly required. The practice of 'topping up the patient' after surgery has pretty much disappeared as a result of the AIDS problem.

With regard to the future, doctors and scientists cannot guarantee that other blood-borne viruses or other dangerous organisms will not one day become transmitted by blood. As we have learned from the AIDS tragedy, we must first be able to isolate the virus before we could institute a reliable way of screening for it in blood. Because of the possibility of new diseases developing in the future, and the very small chance of contracting current diseases from blood transfusions, there will always be some risk associated with receiving blood products. It is important to keep a proper perspective on this. In many cases, the risk from *not* accepting blood when the physician feels it is vitally important may far out-weigh the risk of disease transmission. Each case must be considered individually since no two patient's needs are ever the same. Don't be afraid to discuss your feelings about blood transfusion with your doctor. He or she will understand your reservations and should be prepared to clearly justify the need for blood if it becomes necessary.

Bowel Prep

Before radical prostate surgery, it is important that the bowel be cleansed of feces. During a radical prostatectomy, the rectal wall may be injured, especially if it is difficult to separate the prostate from it. Since feces contain enormous numbers of bacteria, any spillage during surgery may cause an infection.

In order to cleanse the colon before surgery, patients are given a 'bowel prep' (short for bowel preparation). The bowel may be 'prepped' either by drinking large volumes (4 liters) of a specially-prepared salty fluid, or by taking a combination of laxatives and enemas. The bowel preparation is done in the hospital after admission and is prescribed by the surgeon or residents. Some surgeons start their patients on a bowel prep the day before they enter hospital.

Antibiotics

Antibiotics are given to minimize the chances of infection. Some surgeons prescribe oral tablets, beginning a day or two before surgery. Others order intravenous antibiotics to be started just before the operation and to continue for a few days after the surgery. *If you are allergic to any antibiotics, be sure to remind your surgeon or the residents!*

Abdominal Shave

Removal of all the hair on the lower abdomen used to be a routine procedure before an abdominal operation. Recently, however, there has been some evidence to suggest that shaving, unless done just before surgery creates small cuts where bacteria may grow. This, in turn, may lead to an increase of the wound infection rate. Consequently an abdominal shave is not nearly as popular as it used to be and has become a matter of the surgeon's preference. The evidence that it is harmful is not very strong and so you can leave this decision up to your surgeon.

A Visit by the Anesthetist

The evening before your operation you will be visited by an anesthetist. He or she will review your medical history and ask you about prior anesthetic experiences. You are entitled to enquire about the various types of anesthesia which may be suitable for your operation, and you may express your preference.

For radical prostatectomy a general anesthetic is required. For a transurethral prostatectomy, a spinal anesthetic is preferred. Your anesthetist should be able to present the various choices and provide a recommendation of what is best for you.

Chapter 21
Surgical Therapy

TRANSURETHRAL PROSTATECTOMY

If the prostate has enlarged sufficiently to obstruct the bladder, the patient has only a very small opening through which to void, therefore a new passageway for urine must be created. A **transurethral prostatectomy** accomplishes this. The operation can usually be done under a spinal anesthetic, but sometimes a general anesthetic is used. In the operating room the patient is given his anesthetic and placed on a special table. His legs are raised into stirrups and his genitalia cleansed with an antiseptic solution. After covering the patient's legs with sterile drapes, the urologist passes the cystoscope up the urethra (fig 20 & 21). A fibre optic light source and continuous water flow through the instrument are used to ensure a good view.

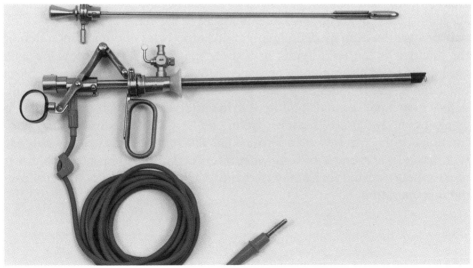

Figure 32. The resectoscope.

The urethra usually allows the cystoscope to pass, but if it does not, metal or plastic tubes may be used to stretch and hold the passageway open. The cutting instrument (resectoscope, fig 32) is inserted and the excess tissue is scraped away from the inside of the prostate with a small wire connected to an electric current. The process is analogous to coring an apple and leaving the surrounding pulp. The scrapings are removed through the resectoscope sheath and the newly-formed channel is cauterized to stop the bleeding. The urine will now pass readily. The fact that at the level of the prostate the normal lining of the urethra has been removed does not seem to be a problem. A catheter is left in the penis and water is continuously irrigated through the bladder to wash out any blood that collects during the first day or two. The catheter is removed once the urine has cleared of blood. The patient usually finds that he is able to void with a strong stream although he may have some irritation for a few days or weeks.

It is rare to note any loss of sexual function other than a marked decrease of the volume of ejaculate during orgasm. This is due to loss of fluid-producing glandular tissue as well as to the permanent opening of the bladder neck which would normally able to close during ejaculation to force the fluid out through the penis. Following prostatectomy, ejaculatory fluid may eject backwards into the bladder and appear in the next urination. This phenomenon is known as **retrograde ejaculation** (fig 33) and is not harmful.

Transurethral prostatectomy is generally safe and well-tolerated. Hospitalization is usually only 3 to 5 days and patients recuperate quite quickly. Heavy lifting and straining must be avoided for at least 6 to 8 weeks after surgery to prevent abrupt pressure increases in the veins of the pelvis which could causebleeding by dislodgement of a blood clot or a scab. Infection of the bladder or the epididymis or testicle may occasionally develop as a complication of transurethral prostatectomy. This is not a serious problem but it can be painful and may require several weeks of antibiotic treatment. A few men have some dribbling of urine after surgery; this may be due to weakness of the control muscle ("sphincter", fig 12) or to involuntary contractions of the irritated bladder muscle. These problems usually subside within weeks or months and only very rarely constitute a chronic problem. It is extremely unusual for a patient to have total loss of urinary control following this operation.

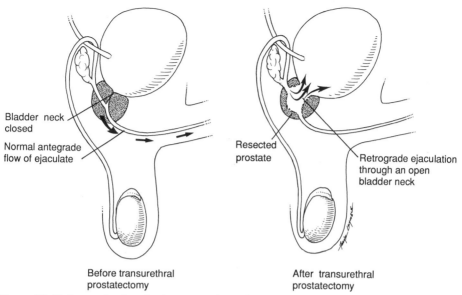

Bladder neck
closed

Normal antegrade
flow of ejaculate

Resected
prostate

Retrograde ejaculation
through an open
bladder neck

Before transurethral
prostatectomy

After transurethral
prostatectomy

Figure 33. Retrograde ejaculation occurring after transurethral prostatectomy.

Chapter 22
Radical Prostatectomy

When a prostate cancer is thought to be confined within the gland, there is a good chance that it can be cured by aggressive treatment. This entails total removal of the prostate or extensive radiation of the area.

A recommendation for total removal of the prostate (radical prostatectomy) is based on several factors. First of all, the tumor must appear confined to the prostate, that is stage A or B. If the stage is more advanced, a radical prostatectomy is unlikely to cure the patient and the risks and problems inherent in the operation cannot be justified. Also, the tumor markers (PSA, PAP) should not be high and the patient must be medically fit to withstand lengthy anesthetic time and surgery. Advanced age is not an absolute **contraindication** (a contraindication is a reason for *not* doing something) to surgery, but unless the patient has a life expectancy of at least 10 years, surgery is not likely to affect his overall survival. Thus, radical prostatectomy is *usually* limited to patients under the age of 70.

When a man discusses the option of radical surgery with his urologist, he will want to know both the benefits and the risks. The potential benefits are obvious in that the cancer could be completely eradicated and the man would be cured of his disease. The risks, or price that he must pay for this, however, may be considerable. These include immediate postoperative complications as well as the long-term complications discussed below.

As an alternative to radical prostatectomy, there is always the option of radiation therapy. Even though it may not offer as high a cure rate as surgery, radiation therapy can significantly increase an individual's life-expectancy.

THE OPERATION

There are two techniques of radical prostatectomy. The most common is called **radical retropubic prostatectomy** and the second **radical perineal prostatectomy**. The latter procedure involves an incision in the perineum (the skin between the scrotum and the anus). The prostate is approached from behind and removed in its entirety. This operation was very popular in the past but it has been supplanted by the retropubic approach which allows access to the lymph nodes as well as to the prostate gland. With the advent of laparoscopic lymph node dissection, some surgeons are again offering this form of surgery. The radical perineal prostatectomy will not be described any further in this book.

Radical Retropubic Prostatectomy

Preparations for surgery are discussed in greater detail in Chapter 20. In essence, however, a man preparing for a radical retropubic prostatectomy should maintain good nutrition, and if he is obese he should try to lose some weight to make both the surgery and postoperative recovery less troublesome. Smokers should quit or cut back to maximize lung performance and lessen chances of lung complications. A wash out of the bowel is done on the day before surgery. This usually involves a limited fluid diet and drinking up to 4 liters of a special solution that cleanses the bowel.

On the day of surgery the patient receives intravenous antibiotics just before the operation. After the general anesthetic, a very fine pressure-sensitive tube is placed in the jugular vein of the neck so that the total blood volume, and heart function can be monitored. Then a catheter is placed into the bladder and an incision made in the lower abdomen from the pubic bone (the bone just above the base of the penis) to the navel. First the lymph nodes that drain the prostate are dissected out and sent to the pathologist for **rush section** (immediate examination). If these lymph nodes are free of cancer, then the prostatectomy can proceed. If the lymph nodes contain enough cancer to be visible by the surgeon in the operating room, the cancer has advanced to the point where a radical prostatectomy is no longer curative and the procedure is abandoned. There is a controversial, 'grey' area, where the lymph nodes are normal size but the 'rush section' pathologist identifies one or a few microscopic areas of cancer within the lymph nodes. In this situation it is difficult to know whether or not to go ahead with the radical prostatectomy or not. Recent evidence suggests that the prostate should be removed with the lymph nodes and hormone-withdrawal therapy (Chapter 26) instituted soon after surgery. Before entering the operating room, it should be clear in both the patient's and surgeon's mind what will be done in any of the possible situations that could be encountered.

After the lymph nodes are removed, the prostate is taken out. The traditional radical prostatectomy involved removal of the prostate and a large amount of the surrounding tissues (wide resection). Within these surrounding tissues are nerves and blood vessels that run alongside the prostate

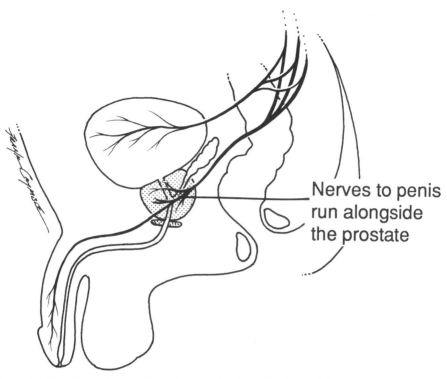

Figure 34. Sideview of normal anatomy prior to radical prostatectomy.

Nerves to penis run alongside the prostate

gland to the shaft of the penis (fig 34). These nerves are vital for erection of the penis. In the classic prostatectomy of the pre-80s era, 80% to 90% of patients lost their ability to attain an erection (that is, became impotent,fig 35). In 1983, a modified technique was introduced by Dr. Patrick Walsh. Walsh's procedure protects the nerves from injury by dissecting between the edge of the prostate and the nerves that run parallel to it (fig 36). This **nerve-sparing prostatectomy** can only be used when the prostate cancer does not extend to the edge of the gland. If there is doubt as to whether or not the entire cancer can be removed, a wider margin must be used which increases the chance of impotence.

In theory, if the nerves are surgically spared then the patients should remain potent. However, for a variety of reasons, potency is preserved for only 70% of patients, the others suffer some loss. Also, if the cancer is more extensive and a wider operation is necessary, only 40% of patients will remain potent. (The options for treatment of impotence are discussed in Chapter 32)

During a radical prostatectomy it is not unusual to lose moderate, or even large quantities of blood from the big veins which run alongside the prostate. While great efforts are made to secure these veins, the patient should be prepared to receive **blood transfusions** during and after surgery if

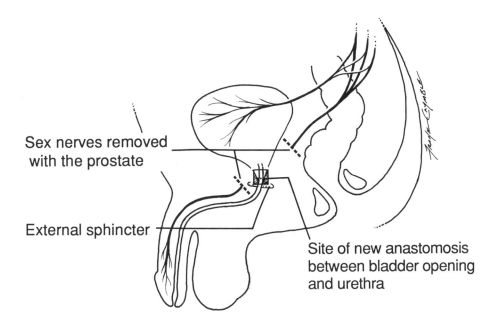

Sex nerves removed
 with the prostate

External sphincter

Site of new anastomosis
between bladder opening
and urethra

Figure 35. The classic radical prostatectomy removes the nerves.

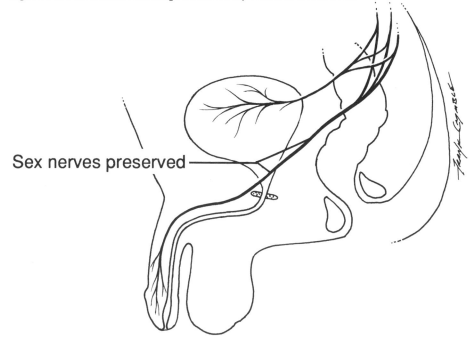

Sex nerves preserved

Figure 36. The nerve-sparing radical prostatectomy.

required. Donation and storage of one's own blood during the weeks before surgery is available at some, but not all, hospitals. This is an issue that a patient should discuss with his surgeon before hospitalization.

Once the prostate has been removed, the bladder is reconnected to the urethra (figs 35 & 36). A catheter (**Foley catheter**) must be left in the bladder for 10 to 20 days to allow the newly formed junction (**anastomosis**) to heal. A small rubber tube is inserted into an opening next to the main incision to drain any blood or urine that might otherwise collect under the wound in the first days after surgery.

The prostate is an integral part of the urinary control mechanism (**continence**) of the male. Once it has been removed, the patient becomes more reliant on the voluntary ('external') sphincter muscles to maintain continence (fig 37). It is common for a patient to dribble some urine involuntarily after removal of the catheter, but in most cases this clears up within a few months or even weeks as the patient learns to control the remaining muscles. Many patients have only mild incontinence, encountered during physical stress such as heavy lifting or coughing. More serious incontinence requiring protective pads is most unusual, and occurs in only 1% to 2% of cases. This complication is discussed in Chapter 33.

The first few days of recovery are marked by pain at the incision, especially on deep breathing or a change of position. Despite the pain, it is very important to get up as early as the day after surgery and begin walking. Even while in bed, the legs must be moved frequently to prevent **blood clots**

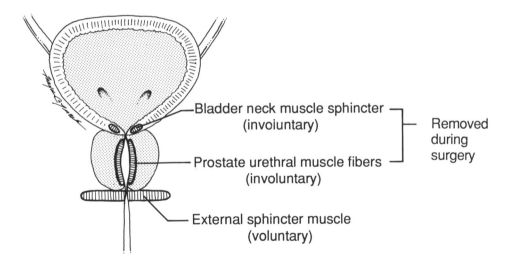

Figure 37. The normal urinary sphincters.

from developing in the leg veins because such clots can travel to the lungs and cause serious complications. Similarly, although it may be painful, it is vital to do frequent deep-breathing exercises to prevent collapse of the lung spaces and the development of **pneumonia**.

Most patients can tolerate small amounts of fluids by mouth as soon as one day after surgery, and a regular diet can usually be resumed by the third postoperative day. Skin sutures or staples are removed on the seventh day and, as mentioned, the catheter and drain are usually removed some time after the tenth day depending on the patient's recovery. It usually takes 6 to 8 weeks before a man recovers his preoperative energy level. It is possible to take on light activities and paperwork within a couple of weeks of surgery, but more vigorous exercise, work, or travel should be avoided for at least two months.

PROCESSING THE SPECIMEN

The diagnosis of cancer is already made when the surgeon decides to operate on a patient. After the surgery, the job of the pathologist is not to tell the surgeon whether or not the patient really had the cancer but to characterize the cancer so that **prognosis** and the need for further treatment can be determined. In fact, the pathologist continues the staging process that the physician began before surgery.

Once the prostate and the cancer it contains has been removed, it becomes a '**specimen**' and is immediately sent from the operating room to the pathology department. The specimen is washed with water, then immersed in formaldehyde for 24 to 48 hours to be 'fixed.' The formaldehyde kills bacteria and cells, and prevents decomposition so it preserves the specimen.

The first part of the pathologist's examination consists of a careful inspection of the specimen, recording the shape, size and position of the abnormalities (fig 38A). A number of slices are made through the prostate, particularly at the level of what feels and looks to be the area of cancerous growth (fig 38B). Representative areas are selected from which small samples are taken for detailed microscopic examination (fig 38C). From these samples the pathologist can determine the extent of cancer spread into and through the prostate capsule. Next, sections are cut from the seminal vesicles and the urethra at both ends of the gland. The remaining tissue is reimmersed in formaldehyde to be stored, in some cases for years, should further examination become necessary.

The selected samples are frozen or embedded in **paraffin** so that they can be sliced thinly enough for microscopic analysis (fig 39A). The thin

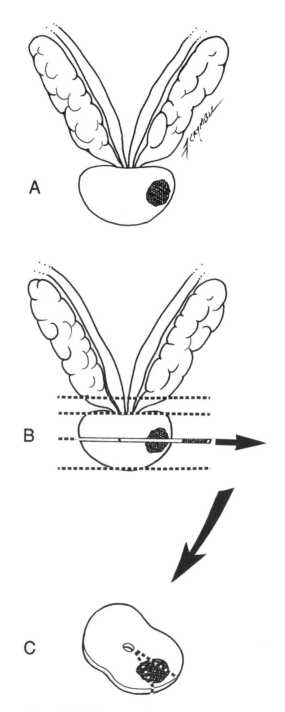

Figure 38 a,b,c. Preparation of pathology specimen.

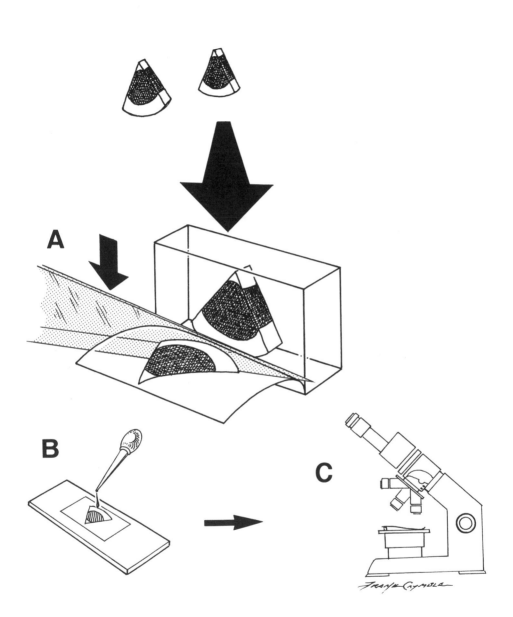

Figure 39 a,b,c. Preparation of paraffin section for microscopic analysis.

83

slices are placed on glass slides and colored with stains to make the structures easier to see (fig 39B). These ultrathin, stained slices of the specimens' representative areas are 'read' by the pathologist. Each slide is examined under the microscope (fig 39C) and the pathologist dictates a report into a tape recorder. The report is typed and becomes part of the patient's permanent record. If the pathologist has questions about the case, it is easy to carry the slides down the hall to the office of a colleague to obtain a second opinion. Once the diagnosis is satisfactory, the findings are relayed.

This process of reviewing the specimen is a complex one which, if it is to be done properly, requires a certain amount of time - in a busy hospital that can mean anywhere from 48 hours to 10 days.

STAGING BY THE PATHOLOGIST

As the surgeon did before the operation, the pathologist attempts to stage the cancer afterwards. While the surgeon had to stage the patient without the benefit of actually having the specimen, the pathologist stages the specimen without having the benefit of seeing the patient! Of course, the pathologist

THE ART OF PATHOLOGY

While most people can accept that medicine is an inexact science, even fully-trained physicians are surprised when they learn that the specialty of **pathology** is also somewhat of an art form.

Being able to distinguish an area of severe dysplasia (abnormal appearing cells that may be precancerous) from an established cancer is one of the 'soft' areas of pathology. The difference comes down to an impression based on the microscopic appearance of a group of cells. Every case is slightly different, so it is impossible to 'go to the books' whenever there is some doubt. Sooner or later, a pathologist (if he or she is worth his or her salt) has to put himself on the line and provide the diagnosis. They who hedge too often find that soon specimens are shunted to their more definitive colleagues, by surgeons unwilling to work with diagnostic uncertainty.

This is not to say that in every case hunches and the pathologist's personality are important to the diagnosis. As in other specialties, as much as 95% of what a pathologist sees is straightforward and not particularly challenging. In those other 5% of situations however, a second pathology opinion may be warranted. One such area is in the determination of whether an area is dysplastic or whether it is a cancer. Another is determining the percentage of tissue that is involved with cancer, and whether a tumor has been completely excised by surgery. When doubt exists, most pathologists will consult their colleagues for another opinion before issuing a final statement. If the treating physician feels that the report remains ambiguous or unsatisfactory, a request may be issued that the tissue specimens and prepared microscopic slides be sent for review by a more experienced uropathologist.

may obtain some information about the patient's status, but in most cases, the **pathological stage** is determined based on the surgical specimen only.

Any spots where the cancer is close to the gland's capsule will be carefully examined to see whether or not the cancer cells are confined to the gland or have broken through.

If the sections show that the **surgical resection margin** (the outer surface of the specimen) has cut across a cancer-containing area, then one must assume that there are still some cancer cells left behind in the body. This is sometimes referred to as **positive resection margins**. Such a situation may necessitate additional treatment, with either radiation or hormones. If, on the other hand, the cancer appears to be completely encased within the specimen (**negative resection margins**) then it is probably completely removed which means that there is a high chance of cure, perhaps in the 70% to 80% range. The missing 20% to 30% represents patients who have undetectable metastases at the time of surgery, or small areas of spread near to, but beyond the margins of the specimen, that could not be identified by either the surgeon or the pathologist.

Chapter 23
Recovering from Surgery

EXTUBATION

During a **general anesthetic**, both sleeping (anesthetic) and paralyzing drugs (muscle relaxants) are given. The former produces unawareness during surgery and the latter relaxes the muscles so the surgeon can get at the area of interest. As the patient is deeply asleep and without muscle control, his breathing must be done for him. To facilitate breathing, shortly after the patient reaches unconsciousness the anesthetist slides a small tube (**endotracheal tube**) through the mouth and into the trachea (fig 40). The endotracheal tube is attached to a ventilator which then moves air in and out of the lungs. During the operation the anesthetist's job is to monitor the ventilator's performance and to be ready to intervene at any moment if problems develop.

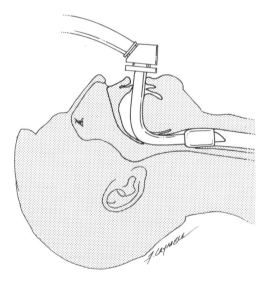

Figure 40. Endotracheal tube.

When the operation is completed and the surgeons are sewing the wound closed, the anesthetist begins to reduce the concentration of anesthetic gas. The patient gradually drifts toward consciousness while the bandages are applied. Breathing, which was done for the patient by the ventilator, becomes spontaneous (the patient takes over). When the anesthetist is convinced that the patient is awake enough to breathe safely on his own, he removes the endotracheal tube from the patient's throat and talks reassuringly to reorient him to the unfamiliar operating room surroundings. Orderlies, doctors and nursing staff shift the patient from the operating table onto a stretcher which carries him down the hall to the recovery room.

NOTIFYING YOUR IMPORTANT OTHER

In most cases, there is someone whom you wish contacted when the operation is finished. It is important that that person's name and phone number be clearly written on the chart and that he or she is standing by awaiting the call. While you are being wheeled to the recovery room, your surgeon is reaching for the phone to contact this person. The surgeon will describe what was found (if that is your wish), and what was done and how the operation went. Rarely, if there is a difficult decision to be made during an operation, the surgeon will 'scrub out' while you are still asleep and contact this person as your 'patient rep' to involve him or her in the decision. Make sure there is only one person to call. The surgeon is not interested in calling a 'board meeting' and does not have time to answer calls from a variety of people, all claiming to be cleared for confidential information about you. It should be clear that the patient representative will act as the sole liaison between family, friends and the surgeon until you are ready to resume that role.

THE RECOVERY ROOM

The anesthetist goes with the patient to the recovery room and stays close by until he is certain that there are no problems. Meanwhile, the surgeon provides the recovery room nurses with a list of orders that cover a variety of areas including directions for pain relief, timing of appropriate blood tests, and instructions for giving antibiotics or other medication.

Most patients can't remember much about their stay in the recovery room, even though they respond appropriately (but slowly) to questions and commands while they are there. Mostly they sleep, groan, or smile bravely after being reassured that their operation is over and that they have survived.

Beyond ensuring that patients are as comfortable as possible, recovery room nurses fulfill two critical roles: they make sure that the anesthetic has been appropriately 'reversed,' and they maintain a vigil for early surgical complications.

Inadequate Reversal

'Reversing' is a term used to describe the procedure of waking a patient after anesthetic. It may be done simply by turning off anesthetic agents (inhaled gases) or by giving **intravenous reversing agents**. Sometimes a combination of methods is used.

Occasionally, a patient who appeared to be waking up adequately, drifts back into a light anesthetic haze in the recovery room and is in danger of suffocation because his *sedated* brain does not recognize his ineffective breathing effort (this does not happen during normal sleep as the *sleeping* brain remains acutely aware of breathing and oxygen levels). Recovery room nurses are on the lookout for 'inadequate reversal' and when they notice it, the patient will be roused by talking, physical stimulation (pinching or some other harmless but annoying act), or by giving certain drugs which supplement the reversal process.

Bleeding

In the recovery room bleeding does not happen often, but when it does, it can be very serious and must be identified quickly. Bleeding at this stage usually means that a tie on a blood vessel has come away, or that a cut blood vessel that was not bleeding during the operation has decided to 'let loose.'

Identifying postoperative bleeding requires skill and experience because it is rarely visible. The bleeding is usually internal and can only be recognized by watching the patient's vital signs (pulse, blood pressure, respiration rate) and the wound area. An unusually high or increasing heart rate may mean that the heart is having to pump faster to provide adequate circulation because there is less blood to go around as a result of hemorrhage. A low blood pressure may mean that the patient is losing blood and doesn't have enough to maintain normal pressure.

In a radical prostatectomy, the surgeon will leave a **drain** in the wound so that normal amounts of fluid and blood may be evacuated. One end of the tube is placed in the surgical area and the other end is brought out through the skin. Some types of drains are connected to a gentle suction pump. An excessive amount of blood coming through the drain is one of the easier ways to identify abnormal postoperative bleeding (this is one of the reasons some surgeons use drains). Bleeding after radical prostatectomy may also be indicated by an abnormally bulging or distended abdomen. In the case of a transurethral prostatectomy, the nurse will watch for abnormal amounts of bleeding through the catheter.

If the recovery room nurse identifies signs of bleeding, the surgeon is called promptly to examine the patient. The surgeon may decide to take the patient back to the operating room and re-anesthetize him. The abdomen will be reopened, the accumulated blood evacuated and the bleeding points tied off. Needless to say, surgeons hate having to do this, but most have learned that it is better to 'bite the bullet' and go back in to deal with this kind of trouble. Excessive bleeding that is not evacuated may eventually stop on its own, but it will leave a large, deep blood clot (**hematoma**) which may delay wound healing and increase the chance of infection.

The amount of time spent in the recovery room varies with the type of operation as well as with hospital policy. In general, however, the patient stays in the recovery area until he no longer needs the one-to-one attention. Some patients remain in the recovery room overnight or longer, if further observation or treatment is warranted. Many hospitals have a policy that a transfer to the Intensive Care Unit be considered if things are still not going well after an overnight stay in the recovery room.

THE WARD

Most patients recovering from major prostate surgery will spend 7 to 14 days on the ward. When departure time finally rolls around, they are usually quite pleased to be saying farewell. A few particulars regarding postoperative ward life deserve mention.

Pain

Pain after surgery is unavoidable. Fortunately, much of it can be controlled with strong **analgesics** (pain killers) available in hospital.

The most common regimen for managing surgical pain in the first few postoperative days is (buttock) injections of a narcotic (*eg* morphine or Demerol™) every three to 4 hours. Don't feel guilty about needing the injections, or fear that you will turn into a drug addict. After all, this is why science developed these medications! Some hospitals are using a new system of providing drugs to patients which is known as PCA or **patient controlled analgesia**. In this system, the patient has a button within reach that he can press when he begins to feel pain. The button activates a pump which delivers a small, preset amount of morphine into the intravenous set, giving immediate pain relief. In this way, the level of pain killer in the blood is kept relatively constant. Studies have shown that patients on the PCA system actually use a lower total amount of narcotic during the postoperative period. Ask your surgeon if PCA is available in your hospital.

As the third or fourth day after surgery passes, the need for strong drugs diminishes. Once eating is resumed, tablet-form pain killers are usually adequate.

Urine Output

An important piece of postoperative information is urine volume. The volume of urine made reflects the amount of fluid and blood in the circulatory system. After major surgery, fluid weeps into the irritated tissues of the pelvis and the amount of fluid in the veins and arteries can drop. This is known as **third space loss**. When third space losses are great, the kidneys try to keep fluids in by reducing urine output. This is fine, up to a point. However, if the circulating blood volume gets too low, the kidneys and other organs become starved of fluid and begin to suffer irreparable damage. By keeping track of the amount of urine made, third space losses can be estimated. If the urine output is too low, more intravenous fluid will be given to compensate for this.

The Patient's Role

You should not get the idea that your postoperative period will be peaceful, and that you will lie in bed attended like a queen bee in a hive. Rather, you may find that your nurses unceremoniously kick you out of bed and force you to walk up and down the halls, even though walking causes you increased pain. They know that there are fewer surgical complications when patients are mobile as soon as possible after surgery. In particular, there is less chance of developing blood clots in the legs and intestinal function is thought to return more promptly in patients who get up and move about.

Deep-breathing exercises are also important: after abdominal and pelvic surgery there is a natural tendency to take shallow breaths because deep breaths hurt. Shallow breathing can cause areas of collapse in the lungs (**atelectasis**) which may cause fever and may lay the foundation for pneumonia. For this reason, patients are asked to force themselves to take three consecutive, painfully deep breaths every 15 minutes when they are awake, for at least the first week following surgery. These exercises should only be done lying flat on the bed as deep breaths in the sitting or standing position can cause a feeling of faintness.

In many hospitals, **physiotherapists** assist with these important breathing exercises. Small plastic bedside devices called **incentive inspirometers**

90

are available to allow the patient to measure his deep breathing efforts.

Going Bonkers

Going a bit nutty after surgery is common. **Postoperative confusion** may occur, most often in patients over the age of 50, and is probably caused by a combination of the stress of surgery, unfamiliar surroundings, pain, anxiety, separation from family, medications, and a disrupted sleep cycle. The symptoms of postoperative confusion include anything from mild disorientation to real hallucinations. Previously placid individuals have been known to become bedpan-throwing menaces. This can be frightening for both the patient and family (and dangerous for staff!). Anyone from grandpa to chief executive can develop postoperative confusion, but a major operation is usually required.

Fortunately, postoperative confusion is temporary. Treatment may include a change of rooms, other medication and occasionally, a brief period of treatment by a psychiatrist. Since serious infection and other medical problems can contribute to postoperative confusion, it is important that these be ruled out. Provided there is no underlying problem however, time may be the most important aspect of treatment. Sooner or later, if the person is otherwise doing well, he will come out of it and may or may not recall this difficult period. Those who do are often quite sheepish about how they behaved and need to be reminded how 'normal' postoperative confusion is.

This simple type of confusion must be differentiated from the disturbance seen in patients who were excessive drinkers before surgery and who develop confusion and other symptoms of alcohol withdrawal during the postoperative period. Such patients may go on to develop **delirium tremens (DTs)** which, unlike simple postoperative confusion, may have serious medical implications.

Stitches

Nowadays, wounds may be closed with either stitches, staples or adhesive tape strips. Stitches and staples may be removed 7 to 10 days after surgery, depending on the site of the operation. In general, stitches or staples left in for more than 7 days serve little purpose and are more likely to leave a visible 'stitch scar.'

A Note About Visitors

Other than winning a lottery, there is little that can compete with a stay in the

91

hospital for bringing friends and relatives out of the woodwork. Depending on your personality and your medical condition after surgery, this may or may not please you. If it does not, the simplest way of avoiding the stress of attending to a steady stream of visitors is simply not announcing to anyone other than your immediate family that you are going in for surgery. Patients may wish to 'be away on a vacation'. For individuals who manage to find out your secret, a 'no visitors policy' (you can say that the surgeon insisted) will be strictly enforced if an order is written in the chart. This can be modified to permit special visits.

GOING HOME

A Departure Checklist

You are bound to have questions about your home rehabilitation and follow-up, so write them down and be prepared to rattle off the list when you see your doctor for the last time in hospital. The moment of discharge always feels like a small victory for any surgeon, and most are in the mood to take a few moments to answer some questions. By keeping a list, you are less likely to leave out an important concern.

Make sure you understand any instructions about temporary limitations of physical activity, discharge medications (make sure appropriate prescriptions are left for you), dressing changes (if any), and follow-up.

You may wish to leave something for the nursing staff, but this is totally voluntary. It is not appropriate to 'tip.' Rather, a box of chocolates or nuts left at the nursing station for the ward staff is always appreciated.

The First three Months

The first 12 weeks at home are a time of major adjustment. It is the rare patient indeed who passes through this phase without significant physical and emotional 'teething' problems. It is a time of adjustment to the trauma of the surgery and the challenge of reintegration into family and work life. Physical problems include intermittent bouts of abdominal pain, constipation, diarrhea, incontinence, hematuria and fatigue, all of which should fade as the 6 to 12 week mark approaches. Constipation and diarrhea may both be treated effectively by fiber supplements such as bran cereal or Metamucil™. Mood swings are common, and the occasional crying jag must be seen as relatively normal.

Timing of the return to work will depend upon the smoothness of the recovery period, and the nature of the patient's occupation. To permit the wound to gain its maximal strength, lifting more than 5 to 10 pounds (the weight of a telephone book!) or straining during the first three months must be avoided and this will influence the timing of a return to work. The person who works at a desk job can expect to return to work within three to 6 weeks of discharge from the hospital. Someone employed in a position requiring stressful physical work will require more time away, or a modification of his job until he is able to begin lifting again. Your physician is in the best position to help you weigh the various influences and with you, plan an appropriate return. As well, your doctor is usually more than happy to provide your employers or insurance people with the necessary documentation needed to protect you during these times.

SURGICAL FOLLOW-UP

A man who undergoes radical prostate surgery should expect to visit his physician often for check-ups (**follow-up**). During the first year he will see a lot of his doctor, regularly every few months, but as time goes by without cancer recurrence, the follow-up examinations will fade to annual visits. Each follow-up visit involves an enquiry into general health, questions concerning the status of urination and a physical examination. The 'physical' includes a digital rectal examination because a cancer which recurs in the prostate bed may be felt through the rectal wall as a vague thickening or a definite nodule. Also, at each visit a blood sample will be taken for a PSA measurement. As a rising PSA level indicates the presence of prostate cancer cells in the body, it may signal a **relapse** well in advance of any other sign. It may take 7 to 10 years for a **recurrence** to become evident, so it is quite important for a man who has had surgery to continue with his annual examinations.

Chapter 24
Surgical Complications

Complications are the problems that can arise during or after an operation. They are more common than one might think, and they vary in significance from minor infections of the surgical wound to catastrophic lethal events.

HOW COMMON ARE COMPLICATIONS?

The public assumes that complications do not arise in the practise of a competent surgeon. Unfortunately, complications are a fact of life in surgery. If a surgeon does enough operations, he will eventually have his share of complications. Surgeons who do major surgery and claim that their patients haven't had any complications are guilty of selective memory.

In major abdominal and pelvic surgery, a surgeon who performs the identical flawless operation on 100 patients will end up with 70 who 'sail through,' 20 who get into minor difficulties, 8 or 9 who develop more serious complications, and one or two patients who develop life-threatening problems. Operations that stand the test of time are those that provide the best results for the greatest percentage of patients. No one can expect an operation to work out perfectly in every instance.

The reasons complications arise are not always clear. Occasionally, fault can be found with the surgeon, the operative procedure or in a physical condition the patient had before the operation, but the common denominator seems to be that peoples' reactions to surgery are unpredictable. The surgical stress that one person tolerates easily may overwhelm another.

Complication rates also vary from surgeon to surgeon. A specialist who does more difficult operations on sicker patients will almost certainly have a higher complication rate than one who does less critical surgery. Likewise, emergency operations are always accompanied by a higher complication rate than are elective, non-emergency procedures because emergency patients are, by definition, already in trouble. They are generally more ill than non-emergency patients, and there is less time to prepare them physically for the stress of surgery.

Nevertheless, given a comparable group of patients with similar sorts of problems, different surgeons will still have different complication rates. It is very much like the varying yield results produced by mutual fund managers. Unlike mutual funds, however, surgeons are not required to publish their complication rates, so the public cannot base a choice of doctors on something as simple as numbers.

In some cases, the differences in complication rates are partly due to technical competence - there is no question that some surgeons are more adept than others due to better natural mechanical ability, wider experience, or a more thorough training. Technical expertise is but a part of the reason why some surgeons have lower complication rates than others. After all, being able to do the operation well should be a *minimum* requirement for an accomplished surgeon.

It is something else, something called **surgical judgment** that, in the final analysis, keeps the patient out of trouble. Part experience and part instinct, surgical judgment is the means by which the surgeon tailors his approach to each patient by choosing one out of a multitude of possible treatment options. The choice is based on an analysis of the patient, the disease, and the surgeon's own experience with similar clinical combinations. In other words, it might best be described as a 'gut feeling' for what he can and cannot do in a particular situation, balanced against the needs of the patient. In some cases it will prevent him from operating altogether, while in others it will lead him to a bold surgical attack.

INFORMED CONSENT?

Should a patient expect to be warned of every possible complication? Lawsuits have been won based on the fact that while the surgeon duly recited a long list of possible complications to a patient before the operation, unfortunately he failed to mention the one in 5000 possibility that the plaintiff actually suffered!

Unfortunately, if surgeons were required to thoroughly describe every possible complication to every patient, not only would they never have time to operate, but patients would be so frightened that many would die needlessly from their diseases after choosing to avoid the risks of surgery.

One only need look in any pharmaceutical book for the complications of aspirin to realize the tremendous variety of problems that can arise from even the most common of treatments. It is well known that in medical studies, a certain percentage of volunteers who receive only placebo pills (simple sugar tablets) instead of the real experimental drug will have to be withdrawn from the study because of the development of side-effects such as headache, nausea, and dizziness. Clearly, the human being is a complex and unpredictable entity. Imagine, then, the range of complications possible after a major operation on the patient's vital organs.

Many of the most common complications have nothing to do with the operation at all. For the elderly, a frequent problem after any surgery is a hip fracture. This usually happens when the individual falls on the way to the bathroom while convalescing from an operation. Unfortunately, for the elderly, hip fractures can be serious and may even result in death. While one must obviously be careful when managing an older patient in the postopera- tive period, should every 70 year-old advised to undergo an operation be warned that he might end up with a broken hip?

The most practical means of managing this dilemma seems to be to avoid the 'laundry list' method of discussing problems in preference to a more thorough discussion of the *realistic* possible complications. In that way, the limited amount of time available can be spent ensuring that the patient fully understands the most likely outcomes, rather than giving an inadequate run-through of a multitude of remote possibilities.

THE COMPLICATIONS

Complications may be classified as being either directly or indirectly related to the operation. If a patient loses her sight after an eye operation, that is a complication directly related to the operation. If the patient were to develop an allergic reaction to the anesthetic used to do the operation, that would be an indirect complication as it had nothing to do with the operation itself, but was only the result of the patient having undergone *an* operation.

Indirect Complications

In the postoperative period, the most common indirect complications in- clude fever, pneumonia, blood clots, transient psychological changes and heart complications.

fever

Post-operative fever is extremely common. It is most often caused by a disorder of the lungs called **atelectasis**. Atelectasis is the collapse of a portion of the air spaces in the lungs, usually caused by a combination of the effect of the inhaled anesthetic gas on lung membranes, and the tendency of patients to take shallow breaths in the postoperative period. During the first few days after abdominal surgery, deep breaths cause movement within the abdominal cavity and this leads to pain. Patients unconsciously limit this pain by taking shallow breaths, thus favouring the development of atelectasis. Atelectasis is treated by postoperative physiotherapy based on deep breathing exercises (patients don't like this because it hurts), and adequate pain control to reduce the need to underbreathe.

Wound infection is another common cause of postoperative fever. However, while fever from atelectasis can appear within hours of an operation, fevers due to common forms of wound infection normally do not occur until at least three days after surgery. Treatment entails opening the wound on the ward (with the help of local anesthetic if needed) to allow any pus to drain. This usually results in rapid resolution of the fever. If the wound is opened properly, antibiotics are rarely needed unless there is significant infection within the surrounding tissues (not common) or if the patient has an abnormal immune system or significant diabetes.

Following transurethral surgery, the bladder may become infected and cause a fever. This usually requires antibiotic treatment until the catheter can be safely removed from the bladder.

pneumonia

Atelectasis may progress to pneumonia (infection of the lungs) if the air spaces are not opened promptly. As well, certain patient characteristics such as smoking, emphysema or bronchitis may increase the likelihood of this complication. Accordingly, the chance of developing pneumonia after surgery varies greatly with age and the patient's general health, from less than 2% for fit individuals to up to 25% for elderly people with preexisting lung disease.

blood clots

Although an effort is made to get patients out of bed and walking as soon as possible after surgery, inevitably, there is a fair bit of lying around during the recovery period. This, combined with the body's response to the stress of surgery, acts to increase the likelihood of the blood clotting in the veins of the legs and pelvis. Patients who have a past history of clots, or particular physical characteristics (obesity, abnormal leg veins) that increase their risk of clots, are given **heparin** (an anticoagulant) before and for a few days after surgery in an attempt to prevent this problem. Some surgeons treat all their cancer patients with anticoagulants but this is far from a universal practise because there are others who feel that the risk of bleeding from anticoagulants outweighs the risk of clotting. Your surgeon will, no doubt, have an opinion on this and it is probably best to accept his or her general practice in this regard. If you have a history of blood clots, however, be sure to bring this to your surgeon's attention because it might be an important reason for you to have anticoagulants.

The real danger of blood clots is not so much the clot in your leg, but that a leg clot will be carried by the blood flow up through the veins into the heart where it is pumped into the lungs and produces what is called a **pulmonary embolus**. Pulmonary emboli cause difficulty breathing and chest pain and, if large enough, can be fatal.

Aside from anticoagulants, early walking and frequent pumping of the calves by pointing and raising the foot can be help to prevent leg clots. A variety of stockings and mechanical calf-pumping machines are also available in some centers.

postoperative psychological changes

As noted earlier, transient psychological changes are common during the postoperative period. They vary from mild to severe disorientation and personality change. Fortunately, they are almost always transient and can be managed with gentle and understanding nursing care. Occasionally, brief psychiatric assistance is needed.

heart complications

Myocardial infarction (MI, heart attack) can occur after any type of stress, and major surgery certainly qualifies as stress. Nevertheless, current methods of preoperative evaluation and anesthetic management during surgery have greatly reduced the rates of MI during and after surgery. Obviously, an individual with a history of heart disease is at increased risk and surgeons tend to be especially careful with such patients, often putting them into the intensive care unit (ICU) or coronary care unit (CCU) if they feel that the patient would benefit from special monitoring equipment during the early postoperative phase.

Direct Complications

Direct complications are those that are specific to the operation. They may occur during the operation itself (intraoperative complications), within a few days of surgery (early complications), or months to years after the operation (late complications).

intraoperative direct complications

These consist mostly of injuries to the organs adjacent to the operating area. For example, a tear may occur in the rectum when the surgeon separates it from the prostate, or the ureters may be injured because they enter the bladder immediately above the prostatic junction. Careful surgeons are keenly aware of the proximity of the rectum and ureters so that such injuries should be uncommon in experienced hands. In difficult cases, however, particularly if the patient has had pelvic surgery in the past, there is a higher risk of damage to these structures.

Excessive bleeding from the veins running along the upper surface of the prostate may constitute another intraoperative complication. In some cases, despite careful attention to these structures, a large amount of blood is lost and transfusions are necessary.

early direct postoperative complications

Early direct postoperative problems develop within a few days of surgery, often before the patient goes home. They specifically relate to the operation that was done. A dreaded example is leakage from the newly healed anastomotic line between the bladder and the urethra (fig 35). An **anastomotic leak** becomes apparent when the Foley catheter is removed from the bladder. Most anastomotic leaks are minor and resolve when the catheter is replaced for several more days to allow complete healing.

late direct postoperative complications

Late direct postoperative complications include impotence, incontinence, and anastomotic stricture. Impotence and incontinence are discussed in depth in later chapters (Chapter 32 & Chapter 33). Depending on the medical center, rates of anastomotic stricture vary from one to 2%. Symptoms of a stricture include increasing difficulty when emptying the bladder. An anastomotic stricture usually requires some minor stretching using a blunt-ended steel probe. This can be done at the office under a local anesthetic or occasionally in the operating room under a brief general anesthetic.

REDUCING THE COMPLICATION RATE

Patients may have some control over the complication rate by choosing a surgeon, deciding on a specific operation and changing some of their own habits.

The Surgeon

Nobody (including the surgeon) knows precisely what a surgeon's complication rate is. Few keep written records of complications in a form that can be updated and reviewed, and fewer still make such information public. Then how can you find a surgeon who has a low complication rate?

Many patients leave the choice of surgeon up to their family practitioner, or make a decision based on discussions with friends. In most cases the family practitioner is in the best position to guide you. Sometimes, however, he or she may may be locked into a particular referral pattern dictated by a restrictive group practice.

Recommendations by friends tend to be based on the quality of the surgeon's bedside manner. You must keep in mind that the best surgeons do not necessarily possess the warmest bedside manners. Bedside manner is, in some cases, a very specialized form of salesmanship and this is not an aspect of surgery that some surgeons care to pursue. Furthermore, busy surgeons are often not particularly interested in becoming friends with their patients. (Most have a hard enough time remaining friends with their own spouses!) Instead, they see their role as being the one who concentrates on getting patients out of trouble so that the patient can go back to his own friends. In order to do this for many patients every day, a detached manner is sometimes the most efficient.

To find the most appropriate surgeon, do what surgeons themselves do when they, or one of their family, needs surgery: they ask the opinion of someone who works directly with the surgeons. This is easy to do in a university teaching hospital. Senior surgical residents (trainees) tend to be brutally honest when evaluating the skills of their mentors and are usually pleased to be asked to give an opinion on such an important matter.

In some hospitals, surgeons are required to defend their complications to their colleagues on a regular basis. These meetings are generally called 'Death and Complication rounds' (D & C rounds) and can sometimes become quite tense affairs if chaired by a tough chief who perceives that a complication was the result of a preventable error of judgment. While a hospital that conducts regular D & C rounds does not necessarily have fewer complications, it certainly speaks of an important commitment to patient care and quality surgery. Finding a surgeon who works at such a hospital is one way of ensuring that there is some measure of local quality control on his activities beyond those required by the country's national professional body.

You can easily find out whether your hospital carries out D & C rounds by contacting the hospital administration or the Chief of Surgery.

The Operation

For any particular disease state, there is usually more than one type of operation that can be used. Each procedure will have its *pros* and *cons*, its advocates and its critics. One operation may give the best cosmetic results but may compromise potential cure. Another may have a potentially higher cure rate but lead to a high complication rate.

SURGICAL RESIDENTS

Many hospitals are affiliated with universities and have a responsibility to teach surgical residents. While patients usually accept that their busy surgeons require the assistance of the residents on the ward, some become anxious when they learn that the residents may participate in and, in some cases, perform their operation.

Some patients insist that the residents not be allowed into the operating room in order to ensure that only the surgeon does the operation. If the surgeon complied with such a request, not only would he jeopardize his university appointment, he would definitely reduce the patient's chances of getting through the operation without a complication! The fact is that most major operations are difficult and dangerous when done by a single surgeon, so the presence of the resident may be critical to the success of the procedure. A major operation is a team effort in which residents and other assistants play important roles.

From the point of view of who does the operation, the to-and-fro between the surgeon and the assistant is so evenly spread that one would be hard-pressed to say who did more of the work. Another interesting fact is that, in some cases, the senior resident actually may be a better technical surgeon than his chief! Residents frequently operate around the clock and have done so for 3 to 8 years. By the time they are nearing the end of their training, some are very skillful indeed.

A more important question than "Who does the operation?" is, "Who is directing the operation?". We believe strongly that if the surgeon is present at the operating table assisting and guiding the resident, the result will be as good or better than if the surgeon had done it all himself. This is the basis of a strong surgical training program, and excellent patient care. The presence of the senior surgeon ensures that mature surgical judgment prevails at important decision points, and that his critical eye sees that all the technical steps are completed accurately.

The bottom line is that you should not be put off by the fact that some of your care is administered by a resident and that he or she may be participating actively in your operation. It is your right, however, to expect close supervision of residents by the staff surgeon in the operating room, and frequent consultation by the residents with the surgeon when difficult decisions must be made on the ward.

DEALING WITH A COMPLICATION

If you suffer a complication following surgery, should you let your original surgeon try to deal with it or should you 'fire' him and get a new surgeon? Changing surgeons after the development of a complication would be appropriate only if there is reason to believe that there has been negligence on the part of the surgeon. As was discussed above, all surgeons encounter complications, and therefore the fact that one has occurred does not necessarily mean that the surgeon did anything wrong. In most cases, it is best to let the original surgeon deal with the problem as he or she is familiar with your disease and your specific anatomy, having already 'been there.'

In some cases, if the complication is an unusual one or particularly difficult to deal with, a surgeon will seek a **second opinion** from an experienced colleague. This can be taken as a sign of the surgeon's desire to obtain the best possible outcome for his patient rather than as an indication of weakness or uncertainty. Such a review should be welcomed by the patient.

If the surgeon does not suggest it, and there is a question of further management of the complication (such as the need for reoperation), it would not be out of line for the patient to request a second opinion.

In general, the more radical the operation, the greater the chance of complications. The chance of cure may be increased as the extent of the operation increases, but only to a certain point, after which the 'cost' begins to outweigh the benefit.

The operation ultimately chosen to deal with a cancer will depend on the grade and stage of the cancer, the patient's wishes, and the surgeon's preference and experience. In general, operations of heroic proportions are usually not warranted except in very unusual circumstances. Do not be afraid to ask your surgeon for a list of alternative operations and by all means feel free to obtain a **second opinion** before making an informed choice.

The Patient

Some patient characteristics are associated with a higher risk of complications: obesity, smoking, old age, malnutrition, a poor ability to fight infection, and illnesses such as heart disease, diabetes, a previous stroke or blood clots.

Obesity increases the difficulty of performing any abdominal operation. It is much harder to see through the wound into the abdomen, and more difficult to expose the area of interest. Tissues in the abdomen of an obese individual are often fatty, making precise cuts and repairs more difficult.

102

After surgery, obese patients tend to have higher rates of pneumonia, wound infections, and blood clots in the legs. Furthermore, if an obese patient develops a complication in the abdomen, it is often detected late simply because of the difficulty in assessing the abdomen.

Patients who smoke, particularly those with smoking-related lung diseases such as chronic bronchitis or emphysema, are susceptible to the development of pneumonia and other lung problems after surgery. Avoiding smoking, even for as little as a few weeks before surgery, may reduce this risk.

SECTION VII:
NON-SURGICAL THERAPY

Chapter 25
Radiation Therapy

Radiation therapy plays two important roles in the treatment of prostate cancer: curative in localized cancer, and palliative in the patient with advanced, incurable disease.

Radiotherapy must be given carefully. It has the potential to be destructive if it is given without forethought. In fact, it is radiation's damaging effect on tissues that makes it so useful: it is used in the hope that the cancer cells will be destroyed, but special precautions must be taken to reduce the damage to the normal cells of the body.

When radiotherapy is being considered, the patient will be seen by a radiation oncologist, a specialist in the use of radiation for cancer treatment. The radiation oncologist will determine if such therapy is appropriate for the patient, prescribe the amount or 'dose' of radiation and the way it is to be given.

Radiation doses are calculated in terms of **centigrays** (**cGy**) or **rads**. The longer the tissue is exposed to radiation, the greater the dose, and the more the damage. Spreading out the dose over a period of days or weeks by giving a small radiation 'exposure' daily reduces damage to normal tissues. Typical doses are between 4000 and 6000 cGy.

HOW DOES RADIATION WORK?

Radiation works by damaging the genetic material (DNA) of cells. When the irradiated cells try to divide, they do not have sufficient undamaged DNA to complete the division, and they die. Cells that divide frequently are easier to kill than those that divide less often. Since cancer cells divide at a faster rate than normal cells, they are more susceptible to the damaging effects of radiation. This is how radiation kills 'selectively.' Of course, even normal cells divide, therefore it is impossible to prevent non-cancerous cells from sustaining some injury.

HOW IS RADIATION GIVEN?

There are two basic methods of giving radiation. The most common is called **external beam radiation**. With this method the radiation is 'shot' toward the patient from a machine much like x-rays for a chest x-ray. A second method consists of placing radioactive substances within the tissue itself. This sounds somewhat barbaric but it is usually well tolerated. This process is known as **interstitial radiation, implantation radiation** or **brachytherapy** and is discussed in more detail below.

Radiation treatment has to be done at a specialized institution with specialized machines, usually in a cancer clinic. It is not something that can be done in a doctor's office because extra protection must be built into a building where radiotherapy is given: the walls of the radiation room are usually lined with lead to prevent radiation scatter. Most radiation suites are located in the basement or ground floor of the building because it is a lot easier to put all that heavy lead in the bottom of the building than up high, so don't expect much of a view when you arrive for treatments.

Modern day external beam radiotherapy is given by a machine called a **linear accelerator** (fig 41). This technology has replaced the older cobalt

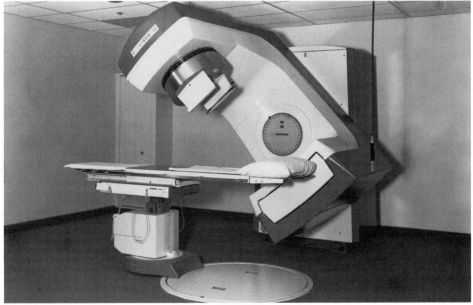

Figure 41. Linear accelerator.

radiation equipment because it has the advantage of being able to focus the radiation more accurately into a discrete target area.

A patient begins treatment with the **treatment simulator**. This is a modified x-ray machine that permits assessment of the patient's abdomen and pelvis. During this procedure a catheter is used to fill the bladder with an x-ray opaque solution that helps to outline the bladder and aid visualization. A small tube is placed in the rectum and filled with air so that the relative position of the rectum can also be seen on the x-ray. In this way the location of the prostate can be mapped out and computers can calculate the exact target coordinates and dosages needed to strike the prostate while avoiding the rectum and the bladder. This *individualized* treatment planning is essential because the location of the prostate varies widely from one patient to another. At the conclusion of **treatment planning,** marks are made on the abdomen with indelible ink (**tattoo**) so that the patient can be positioned exactly the same way each time he returns for a treatment.

The total dose of radiation prescribed for a patient is not given all at once. Rather, it is split into a number of smaller doses in order to minimize side-effects. The patient visits the radiation clinic 4 or 5 days a week for 4 to 6 weeks. He takes off his outer clothing and lies on his back while the machine is aligned. Each session takes 3 to 4 minutes and is absolutely painless. During the session, the technicians who give the treatments retreat behind a leaded glass window for their own protection. If the patient has any concerns during the treatment all he need do is raise a hand and the technician will respond immediately.

For the first week of radiotherapy the patient notices few, if any, effects. However, after several weeks he will feel a growing sense of fatigue. There may be some discomfort in the rectum or bladder, but this can be readily controlled by suppositories or medication. Occasionally a patient will develop some diarrhea and an urge to urinate frequently. For almost everyone, the rectal and bladder symptoms fortunately disappear within the first month or two after the completion of radiation therapy.

Radiation patients should be aware that their ability to attain normal erections may be affected. Overall, 50% to 60% of patients will permanently lose erectile function. It may not be a total loss of erections and it may respond to some simple measures which are outlined in chapter 32.

FOLLOW-UP

The tumor-eradicating effects of radiation may take one or even two years to become fully evident. The follow-up routine is similar to that of the patient who undergoes surgery. A man who has completed radiation therapy must visit the clinic or physician's office every three months for the first year and every 6 months for the second year. During each visit the physician will ask questions and do a rectal examination. Blood will be taken for a PSA test. If the cancer is responding to radiation therapy, the local lump of tumor in the prostate should shrink and become softer as time passes. The PSA level, which was probably high, would return to normal and the symptoms caused by blockage of the bladder by the enlarged prostate cancer should diminish. If these symptoms do not improve, or if they worsen, it is important that the patient let his physician know.

RADIATION TO OTHER PARTS OF THE BODY

If cancer cells have spread to other parts of the body (metastases), radiation therapy may be applied directly to these areas. For example, if a cancer metastasis in a bone is causing pain or if a tumor near the spinal cord presses on nerves and causes loss of sensation and muscle weakness (Chapter 30), then radiation can be aimed directly at these areas. The resulting shrinkage of the metastasis is usually quite rapid, accompanied by a relief from the symptoms in a few days.

OTHER TECHNIQUES OF RADIOTHERAPY

In the early days of prostate radiation therapy, radiotherapists and urologists felt that external beam radiation carried an excessively high risk of damaging the adjacent bladder and rectum. For this reason they used a technique known as **interstitial radiotherapy** (**implantation radiotherapy** or **brachytherapy**). Unlike the linear accelerator, which sends the radiation beam from the outside (external beam), interstitial therapy involves implanting radioactive 'seeds' directly into the prostate. Interstitial radiation does not have to be shot through delicate normal tissues that must be protected. This form of internal radiation therapy is very effective because it allows for the application of much higher radiation doses than can be used with external sources.

Many different types of radioactive sources have been used for interstitial radiotherapy: radium, gold grains, iridium, and iodine 'seeds,' to name just a few. Implantation of the radioactive sources requires surgery and anesthesia. An incision is made in the lower abdomen and the pelvic lymph nodes are sampled and sent for pathology assessment. Hollow needles are inserted through the skin behind the base of the scrotum into the prostate and the needles are guided by a finger in the rectum. The radioactive 'seeds' are implanted through these hollow needles. It is critical that the 'seeds' be distributed throughout the gland in a predetermined pattern so as to distribute the radiation evenly.

Complications from interstitial radiation are usually due to the pelvic lymph node dissection, but impotence and incontinence may also occur. Since the development of accurate external beam machines, brachytherapy is no longer widely used.

Chapter 26
Hormone-withdrawal Therapy

The prostate gland is sensitive to the body's sex hormone levels. From the time of puberty, prostate cells divide and grow under the influence of the male hormone **testosterone** which is produced primarily by specialized cells in the testicles. When cancer cells develop, they too require testosterone for continued growth. In the 1940s, a Nobel Prize-winning discovery confirmed that 'withdrawal' of the male hormone from the body by surgical castration (removal of the testicles) leads to destruction of many of the cancer cells and thus a decrease in the size of the prostate cancer. In other words, if testosterone is removed from the body's circulation, prostate cancer cells are unable to thrive. This discovery led to the treatment of advanced cancer by surgical and medical means of removing testosterone from the body ('**hormone manipulation**'). In at least 85% of cases there is a response to this form of therapy.

After removal of his testosterone, it is not unusual for a man to have symptoms similar to the female menopause, such as hot flushes and mood changes. There are medications available to control these side-effects should they become serious enough to affect a patient's quality of life. Castrated men will have a marked decline of their sexual desires ('libido') and will become impotent (unable to attain an erection). They do not notice any significant change in their other 'maleness' characteristics such as hair patterns, and voice.

SURGICAL HORMONE MANIPULATION

Castration

Surgical castration (**orchidectomy** or **orchiectomy**) is so effective that it is the standard against which all other forms of male hormone withdrawal must be measured. The operation to remove the testicles from the scrotum is quite straight-forward and well-tolerated. It can be done under a local anesthetic, a spinal anesthetic and occasionally, with intravenous sedation to supplement the procedure. The operation is performed through an incision in the middle of the scrotum. The spermatic cords, which contain the vas deferens, blood vessels and nerves (figs 7 & 8), are cut just above the testicles which are then removed. When the scrotum is healed, the space where the testicles had been shrinks somewhat and the individual may feel small lumps which are actually scars at the ends of the cut spermatic cords. If a patient is concerned about the cosmetic aspects or if he is psychologically upset by the 'empty' scrotum, then artificial testes (prostheses) may be inserted.

Surgical castration has very few complications. Postoperative pain is minimal. Bleeding may cause swelling of the scrotum which can be uncomfortable for a few weeks until the blood is reabsorbed. Infection in the incision can occur, as with any type of surgery, but recuperation is normally quite straightforward. When prosthetic testicles are inserted, infection is a rare complication. Antibiotics are often given before and after the operation to minimize the chances of infection, but if an infection does occur the prostheses may have to be removed. After routine surgical castration, most patients go home the same or the next day.

MEDICAL (NON-SURGICAL) HORMONE WITHDRAWAL

Because many men find the concept of surgical castration difficult to accept, urologists have sought alternative means of eliminating the male hormone from the body.

Estrogen Therapy

The first form of so-called 'medical castration' involved the daily administration of the female hormone, estrogen. There are many formulations of estrogen on the market but the most common one is diethylstilboestrol (DES). This drug acts by shutting off the brain's production of the hormone GnRH (gonadotropin releasing hormone) also called LHRH (leuteinizing hormone releasing hormone). This hormone's normal function is to stimulate the pituitary gland to produce leuteinizing hormone (LH), which in turn stimulates testosterone production by the testicles. Thus estrogen administration causes a cascade of effects that ultimately reduces the formation of testosterone by the testicles (fig 42). Although estrogen is effective and relatively cheap, it does have significant side-effects. Besides decreasing male libido and depressing sexual function, it causes swelling of the breasts (gynecomastia). This complication may be prevented by the prior adminis-

110

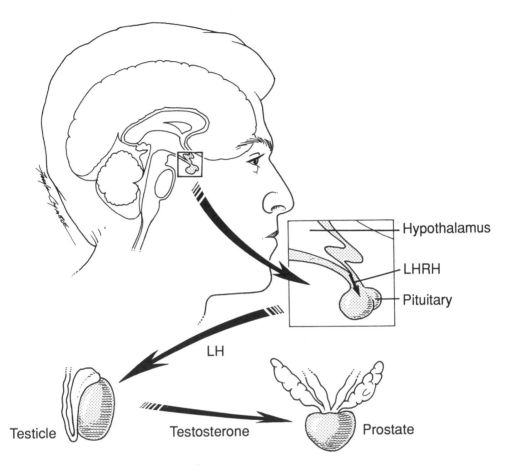

Figure 42. The normal production line of testosterone.

tration of a single dose of radiation to the breast area. Estrogen can also lead to fluid retention with the possibility of weight gain, leg swelling and heart failure. Blood clots may develop in the legs and in some cases travel to the lungs causing extensive, and sometimes life-threatening damage. Finally, estrogen therapy can lead to an increased incidence of heart complications, such as heart attack and stroke. For these reasons and because of the development of safer, alternative drugs, estrogen has lost much of its popularity for the management of prostate cancer.

Non-estrogen Medical Therapy

Because of the complications associated with estrogens pharmaceutical companies have made a great effort to develop and produce alternatives to surgical orchidectomy or estrogen therapy. These drugs act at various levels along the production line of serum testosterone (fig 42). They block either the testicular production of testosterone or the action of testosterone on the prostate cells. Either way, the end point of treatment is the same: the cancer cells as well as the normal hormone-sensitive prostatic cells are deprived of their major growth stimulus.

The selection of the particular means of withdrawing hormones from an individual's body will vary from one institution to another. As well, both the physician's experience and the patient's response to medication play major roles.

Antiandrogens

Antiandrogens block the action of testosterone at the prostate cell level. There are several types currently available for treating prostate cancer.

The first of these is related to the female sex hormone progesterone and there are two of this type, megestrol acetate and cyproterone acetate. They are taken orally on a daily basis and can be given along with a very low dose of estrogen (DES) which enhances their activity. Using these drugs, the effects of surgical castration can be mimicked quite closely and rapidly. Their effects are detectable within a few days of initiating therapy. However, these drugs too, have side-effects. The most prominent are impotence and loss of libido, shortness of breath on exertion, generalized fatigue, nipple tenderness and slight gynecomastia, and a risk, though low, of blood clots and heart disease. They are also expensive.

The second type of antiandrogen does not have a direct effect on the hormones produced by the brain, but acts strongly at the prostate cell level (fig 42) to block the effect of testosterone on the prostate cells. It does not affect testicular production of hormone and thus does not reduce the level of testosterone in the blood. Examples of drugs in this class are flutamide and nilutamide.

When used as the only form of therapy, these drugs may preserve sexual libido and potency by actually elevating the patient's production of serum testosterone (the brain receives a 'message' from the prostate that it is lacking testosterone and steps up production in an attempt to overcome the block). Unfortunately, this rise in testosterone may also stimulate the cancer to grow more quickly, so that these drugs must be given in combination with another form of hormone withdrawal such as surgical castration or an LHRH agonist (see below). Other side-effects include breast enlargement (gynecomastia), diarrhea, nausea and vomiting. These drugs too, are expensive.

LHRH agonists

Another group of medications, called the LHRH agonists, eliminate the body's production of testosterone. These include leuprolide, goserelin, and buserelin. Originally these drugs had to be administered by a daily injection, but now they are available in a 'depot' form that can be injected under the skin on a once-a-month basis. When used alone, these drugs very effectively interrupt the normal production of serum testosterone. When treatment is first begun, there is a transient rise of the serum testosterone which may unfortunately cause a transient worsening of the disease. This 'testosterone surge' may be blocked by co-administering an antiandrogen, at least for the first month or two of therapy. LHRH agonists produce few side-effects except for hot flushes and other menopause-like symptoms. The flushes can be prevented by adding a small amount of the antiandrogen, cyproterone acetate.

Ketoconazole

Ketoconazole is another drug which may be used for the treatment of prostate cancer. This drug is actually available on the market for use as an antifungal agent but it also happens to work very quickly and directly at the level of the testicle to shut off the production of testosterone. This almost instantaneous elimination of testosterone is useful for the treatment of a patient with a cancerous blockage of the urinary channel, kidneys or spinal cord. Unfortunately, its usefulness is limited by significant side-effects such as stomach upset, and by the fact that the patient must take the drug meticulously 'around-the-clock'. Newer derivatives of this medication that can overcome these limitations are now being developed.

INTERMITTENT THERAPY

An innovative approach to hormone-withdrawal therapy for prostate cancer involves a technique called intermittent therapy. If a man is keen on maintaining his sexual function for at least part of his treatment period, then it is possible to transiently lower his serum testosterone to castration levels by using reversible drugs, such as cyproterone acetate. It is known that this drug

IPG RECOMMENDATIONS FOR HORMONE THERAPY

All of the medical alternatives to surgical castration reduce equally the influence of testosterone on prostate cancer cells. There have been some optimistic claims that the combination of surgical castration with antiandrogen drugs may induce longer remissions and even cures. This issue has now been studied in several centers around the world. Although some investigators have assigned minor advantages to the combined treatment, generally the differences in the degree of response have been small and variable. It may be worth to remember the old expression: " For a difference to be a difference it must make a difference."

For the present, a man who is a candidate for hormone-withdrawal therapy should first give serious consideration to surgical castration. If he wishes to forego or delay this form of therapy, then the option of a medical alternative is available. He could start on one, or a combination, of the above described drugs and continue as long as he tolerates them and can afford to pay for them. On the other hand, if he has significant side-effects from the drugs, then he should consider undergoing surgical castration and discontinuing the drugs.

acts very quickly to lower the testosterone level and to achieve remission of the disease. Once the patient has been on drug treatment for 6 or 8 months, his tumor markers have stabilized, and he is without symptoms, the drugs can be stopped to allow his serum testosterone level to return to normal. It takes about two months for him to recover sexual function. The patient must then be medically followed extremely carefully, and his PSA measured monthly, for it is certain that the tumor will reactivate in the presence of testosterone. It may be as long as 6 months before it becomes necessary to reinstitute therapy. In the meanwhile the patient can have normal sexual function. If all goes well, his prostate cancer will respond again to a repeat androgen withdrawal. This form of intermittent hormone therapy, or 'cycling' therapy, is innovative but not widely practiced. It is still being studied in animal model systems and should be considered somewhat risky and experimental. Patient studies are currently being designed to compare this form of therapy to the more standard approach of continuous hormone withdrawal.

AN IMPORTANT LAST WORD ON
HORMONE-WITHDRAWAL THERAPY

Hormone-withdrawal therapy does not cure prostate cancer. The reasons for this are still conjectural. It is possible that in the absence of male sex hormone some cancer cells die while others go into a dormant state. The dormant cells, and perhaps some cancer cells which were never dependent on serum testosterone, continue to grow despite hormone deprivation. Eventually they take over and repopulate the prostate and metastatic sites with what are known as *hormone-resistant* cancer cells. The ideal method of controlling such cells is not clear, but several options are discussed in subsequent chapters.

Chapter 27
Chemotherapy & New Treatment Approaches

CHEMOTHERAPY

Chemotherapy is the use of drugs to fight cancer cells directly. Unfortunately, the cells that cause prostate cancer are not very responsive to chemotherapy. Various agents used alone or in combinations have failed to increase patients' survival. An additional problem is the fact that the typical prostate cancer patient is elderly and may not be able to tolerate the side-effects of chemotherapeutic drugs. Chemotherapy may help some individuals with metastatic cancer (about 1/3 of cases) who receive temporary pain relief before succumbing to their disease.

Unlike other cancers which are readily treatable by chemotherapy, in prostate cancer chemotherapy is usually reserved for patients who already have extensive metastases and are beyond cure. This does not mean that only metastatic cancer is treated by chemotherapy, nor does it mean that when chemotherapy is used, the person is beyond cure. There may be a role for chemotherapy during the earlier stages of prostate cancer. Proponents of early use of chemotherapy suggest that hormone-resistant cells may be present in the cancer when the patient is first diagnosed, so that both a hormone-withdrawal treatment and a chemotherapeutic treatment should be initiated simultaneously to try to destroy both types of cells. Unfortunately, studies have not proven that this combination approach is any better than hormone-withdrawal therapy alone. This may be due to the current lack of a highly potent chemotherapy drug for prostate cancer. Should a chemotherapy drug that works be identified, it would be reasonable to consider routine integration of such a drug into a hormone-withdrawal program early in the course of treatment.

Estracyt™ is a combination of an estrogen (female hormone) and a chemotherapeutic drug. The two are combined on the theory that the estrogen will suppress normal testosterone production while the chemotherapeutic component attacks the cancer cells. To date, the effect of Estracyt™ seems equivalent to conventional estrogen therapy. This agent may be of some use to patients who have had relapses after more traditional hormone-withdrawal therapy. Of note, it is expensive and has some potentially serious side-effects.

NEW TREATMENT APPROACHES

Two new drugs have become available to the patient who has relapsed after traditional hormone-withdrawal therapy and is suffering from widespread bone pain. Both are designed to treat the bone metastases directly. One is a diphosphonate drug known to block the activity of normal bone cells. It has proven to be particularly helpful to patients during the last few months of life, who no longer respond to maximum pain-relief treatment.

The second drug is a radioactive material called strontium, which is injected intravenously and goes directly to the bone. It concentrates itself in the bone metastases and destroys many of the cells, shrinks the bone tumor and reduces the pain. It too, is expensive and is generally reserved for patients who are in pain and at the terminal stage of their cancer. There are side-effects to this drug and limitations to its use, both of which should be discussed with the treating physician.

ON THE HORIZON

The field of immunotherapy which includes the development of antibodies to cancer cells, holds great promise for the future treatment of prostate cancer. Such antibodies, when injected into the blood stream, would exclusively target prostate cancer cells. If scientists could then link a cancer-killing substance to this antibody, an extremely effective and specific treatment would be created. Currently there are many technical problems with this scheme, including the difficulty of developing a highly selective antibody, an effective killing agent, and the means of coupling the two together.

It is known that cancer cells, like normal cells, produce growth factors that stimulate both cancer cells and normal cells to grow and to divide. In response to these growth factors, complex genetic messages are turned on and off during the process of either normal or abnormal cell division. Theoretically, stopping cancer cell division would prevent tumor growth or metastasis. Researchers are investigating the means of controlling the interactions between the genetic messages and the growth factors. These types of agents are still experimental and probably years away from being generally available.

SECTION VIII:
TREATMENT OF ADVANCED DISEASE

Chapter 28
Adjuvant and Neoadjuvant Therapy

THE CONCEPT OF ADJUVANT THERAPY

Adjuvant therapy is treatment given in addition to a potentially curative operation for cancer, in the hope that it will enhance the benefit of the operation. This is different from the treatments given after an operation where the surgeon did not feel that all the cancer was removed. By accepting a course of adjuvant therapy after a potentially curative operation, the patient is 'taking out an insurance policy' against cancer recurrence. He is doing everything he can to maximize his chance of a cure.

It is important to understand the term 'potentially curable.' One never knows whether or not the patient will be cured by a cancer operation, even if it goes without a hitch, and even if the cancer appears to have been totally removed. This is one of the frustrating problems of cancer surgery. There may be tiny, unseen cancer cells left behind in the area of the primary cancer, or growing elsewhere as tiny metastases. Only time can tell whether or not the operation was truly curative.

It is the knowledge that microscopic cancer deposits can be left behind that has fueled the search for effective adjuvant treatments. The question has been: "What else can we do *now* to destroy any microscopic deposits that might remain?"

*Neo*adjuvant therapy is given *before* the surgery; the reasoning being that the tumour will shrink and be more easily and completely removed. Theoretically at least, any microscopic metastases will be destroyed as well. There is some evidence that neoadjuvant therapy can 'down-stage' a cancer, reduce the pathological stage before surgery.

118

WHO BENEFITS FROM ADJUVANT THERAPY?

People with stage A1 or B1 prostate cancer have at least an 85% chance of survival after surgery alone. These patients are normally not referred for adjuvant therapy. Why not have the additional treatment anyway if it might make a difference for the remaining 15% who are not cured by surgery? The reason is that like other treatments, there is a 'price to pay' for adjuvant therapy. The hormones and radiation used as adjuvant treatment have side-effects, and so the 'cost-benefit ratio' is too high for patients who already have a good chance of being cured. In proportion to the number of patients who may benefit, too many cured patients would suffer the side-effects from adjuvant therapy.

Adjuvant treatment is more appropriate to higher stages of disease where there is doubt whether the cancer is totally removed. If a patient has a stage A2 or B2 cancer then there is roughly a 50:50 chance of some tumor being left behind by the surgery. Within 10 years, as many as 35% of these men will suffer a pelvic recurrence of their prostate cancer. For this group, adjuvant therapy makes sense. Radiation treatment to the surgical field, or hormone withdrawal treatments for 6 to 12 months after a potentially curative surgery, *may* reduce these recurrence rates to less than 5%.

Stage D disease is already so advanced that complete surgical removal of the cancer is not possible. Any radiation or hormone treatment given in this setting, in addition to surgery, is called palliative therapy rather than adjuvant therapy.

THE TIMING OF ADJUVANT THERAPY

Animal experiments and clinical data from other cancers indicate that there is an advantage to be had from earlier rather than later adjuvant treatment of a patient who has microscopic spread of cancer. Theoretically, if only a few cells have spread from the main bulk of the cancer, then therapy aimed at the entire body (such as hormone withdrawal, chemotherapy, or perhaps immunotherapy in the future), would destroy those few cells. Once the cancer cells build up and become bulkier growths, then the odds of eliminating all of them diminish. As prostate cancer cells grow, they gradually mutate, change, and become less susceptible to hormone withdrawal, radiation or chemotherapy, permitting them to survive, recover and to multiply. For these reasons, it is thought that adjuvant therapy, if given, should be delivered soon after surgical treatment. Adjuvant therapy research programs at most universities request that patients be enrolled in the study and begin receiving adjuvant treatment within 6 weeks of surgery.

Chapter 29

Hormone-resistant Cancer

Hormone-withdrawal therapy is not a permanent cure for prostate cancer. While most of the cancer cells will die and disappear during treatment, some will remain, eventually to grow again and become **hormone-independent**. This process of regrowth takes an average of 24 months, although some people may become resistant to hormone reduction treatment quickly while others may thrive for years. Once hormone independence has taken place, the cancer becomes a difficult disease to treat. Currently, there is no consensus on the best form of therapy when this happens.

Just because the cancer develops hormone independence, as signalled by the development of 'local,' pelvic symptoms (*eg* urine or kidney blockage, bone pain) or a rising serum PSA, it does not necessarily follow that urgent treatment is needed. If a patient who has had surgical castration is found to have a rising PSA level but no other symptoms, then he may be followed closely without further treatment. On the other hand, if someone who has had hormone withdrawal develops severe pain in his bones from metastases, or other symptoms of recurrent cancer, he should be treated again with a secondary form of therapy (see below). A patient should consider very carefully and discuss with his physician whether or not further treatment should be instituted right away or delayed until the symptoms of metastatic disease become significant.

SECONDARY THERAPY

Secondary therapy is the term used to describe treatment that follows the failure of a first form of therapy.

Radiation Therapy

Radiation therapy may be useful for someone with locally-recurrent or metastatic disease who has been treated with hormone withdrawal but has not been irradiated. A patient with hormone-independent cancer who is having difficulties due to partial or complete blockage of urination, may be well-treated by radiation therapy directed at the prostate to shrink it enough to relieve the blockage. Painful bone metastases may be treated similarly. Of course, all potential benefits of radiation must be weighed against the side-effects of therapy (Chapter 25).

Additional Hormone Suppression

Before secondary therapy is begun, the serum testosterone level should be measured. If testosterone production has been suppressed incompletely, for whatever reason, then a different form of hormone withdrawal should be tried. For example, if an individual has been taking estrogen tablets or an antiandrogen, then surgical castration could be considered. This can provide transient relief of symptoms in about 25% of cases. If, on the other hand, a man's serum testosterone level has been well suppressed, such as after surgical castration or administration of a LHRH analogue alone, then an antiandrogen that works at the cellular level can be started. A response rate of 10% can be anticipated in this situation (10% of patients will improve).

Chemotherapy

The only other secondary treatment alternative to hormone withdrawal is chemotherapy. As previously mentioned, there is no chemotherapeutic agent that is consistently effective against prostate cancer (Chapter 27). Currently, most drugs lead to a positive response in about 15% of patients, and the response is usually short-lived. A patient must carefully consider the risks of chemotherapy (including anemia and loss of infection fighting ability) against the low potential for benefit. This decision should be discussed carefully with the treating physician.

Chapter 30

Emergencies

Emergency situations may arise for patients who have prostate cancer. Occasionally, the emergency may be the first evidence of trouble. Problems can include blockage of the urethra, blockage of the kidneys, bleeding from the prostate, pressure on the spinal cord and weakening of bones to the point of fracture.

BLOCKAGE OF THE URETERS

If the cancer in the prostate grows towards the base of the bladder, it may impinge on the ureters, the tubes that bring the urine from the kidneys to the bladder. There are two ureters, one from each kidney. Obstruction may affect only one ureter or, more seriously, both (figs 13 & 43). If only one

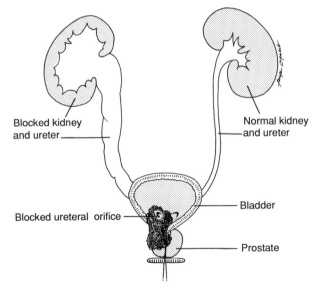

Figure 43. Prostate cancer blocking the right ureter and kidney.

ureter becomes blocked by cancer, it may go unnoticed for many months or even years. Gradually, however, the blocked kidney will be silently destroyed. Accordingly, an obstruction of the ureter must be dealt with on an urgent basis. If both ureters are blocked, both kidneys will fail and death will ensue if treatment is not provided immediately.

In some cases of ureter blockage, one can argue for no treatment. If a patient has advanced, terminal cancer and both ureters are obstructed, nonaggressive treatment may be wise and kind. Death from obstruction of both ureters (kidney failure) is quiet and painless. If, on the other hand, someone is just discovered to have prostate cancer and has one or both kidneys obstructed, then aggressive treatment is usually warranted. Either hormone-withdrawal treatment by surgery or medication should begin right away. Radiation therapy to the area of the prostate and ureters where the blockage has occurred may also be worthwhile. Most patients who have obstructed ureters and who are treated primarily with hormone-withdrawal therapy and radiation therapy will respond well.

Cystoscopy is used to assess the prostate and the ureters. During cystoscopy, dye can be injected into the ureters to delineate the exact location of the blockage. Other common causes of kidney failure must be ruled out: necessary tests include blood tests to measure kidney function, an ultrasound of the abdomen (fig 22), and possibly a CT scan of the abdomen and pelvis (fig 25).

BLOCKAGE OF THE OUTLET OF THE BLADDER

If the cancer in the prostate gland grows inward and impinges on the urethra or urinary channel then partial or total blockage of the bladder can occur (figs 13 & 43). This may develop slowly, with the patient gradually noticing less and less emptying of his bladder, or it may occur suddenly. In both circumstances, treatment involves the insertion of a catheter through the penile urethra into the bladder. If the obstruction will not permit the passage of the catheter through the penis, then a small tube may be inserted through the skin of the lower abdomen into the bladder to drain the urine (suprapubic catheter). This is a relatively simple procedure that can be done under local anesthetic in the Emergency Department or the doctor's office.

If the patient's prostate cancer was not diagnosed before, he will have to undergo transurethral resection of the prostate (with careful examination of the tissue) plus the usual tests. If the cancer is confirmed, staging and appropriate therapy is instituted.

BLEEDING FROM THE PROSTATE

Occasionally, a blood vessel in the prostate or urethra will burst as a result of the growth of the cancer, leading to a sudden hemorrhage into the urine. This is rarely life-threatening, but a fair bit of bleeding can occur and clots which form in the bladder can lead to obstruction of the urethra and severe pain. This is most unpleasant for the patient and needs to be treated urgently by insertion of a catheter into the bladder. The clots can then be washed out through the catheter by an 'irrigation,' or rinse, which stops the bleeding. Occasionally the bleeding continues and a transurethral operation must be done to resect or remove some of the prostatic tissue and cauterize the bleeding vessels. If the patient's prostate cancer was not diagnosed before, and cancer is confirmed by this surgery, the cancer can then be properly staged and appropriate therapy instituted.

PRESSURE ON THE SPINAL CORD

If the prostate cancer has metastasized to the bones of the spine, a mass may develop that impinges on the spinal cord or the nerves leading from it (fig 44). More commonly, this affects the lower spinal cord but any part of the spine may be involved. The symptoms of **spinal cord compression** may develop quickly or over a number of months. Initial symptoms include loss

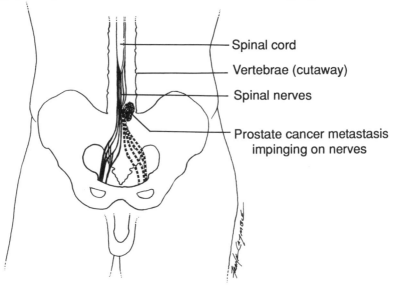

Spinal cord

Vertebrae (cutaway)

Spinal nerves

Prostate cancer metastasis impinging on nerves

Figure 44. Spinal cord compression caused by metastatic prostate cancer.

of sensation, numbness or tingling, weakness in the legs or feet, complete paralysis on one or both sides of the body, loss of bowel or bladder control, or severe pain in the back. By examining the patient carefully, the physician can determine the level of the spinal cord blockage. An exact characterization of the cancerous deposits can be determined by a CT scan of the spine, magnetic resonance imaging (MRI), or a **myelogram**. A myelogram is an x-ray in which dye is injected into the fluid around the spinal cord through a needle inserted in the back. It is a 20 to 30 minute procedure done in the x-ray department by a trained radiologist. A local anesthetic is given to minimize the discomfort associated with needle placement, and some patients will have a transient headache afterwards. Myelograms are being used less often now because of the accuracy, safety, and lesser discomfort of CT scans and MRI.

Initial treatment of spinal cord compression involves giving drugs to shrink any swelling contributing to the blockage. Occasionally, an operation to decompress the spinal cord may be necessary. Radiation therapy to the area should be started promptly so as to restore nerve function. Hormone-withdrawal therapy should begin if the patient has not yet been castrated.

If the spinal cord is blocked at a low level, the only nerves involved may be those leading to the bowel and the bladder. In this case, the individual will be constipated and unable to pass water and may be numb in the anal and scrotal regions. Though this is very frightening for most people, prompt treatment will lead to total or near total eradication of symptoms.

WEAKENING OF THE BONES

When a cancer metastasizes to the bony skeleton it weakens the bone and predisposes it to fracturing. A break through a metastatic deposit is known as a **pathologic fracture**. This area should be irradiated and may require an operation to insert a metal plate or a rod into the bone to secure and encourage whatever healing may be possible. Unfortunately, the bone is often unable to heal naturally because of the cancer, especially if the person has already been treated and has hormone-independent cancer. If a man is diagnosed as having metastatic prostate cancer he should be aware that his bones are weak and he should try to avoid trauma. The most common areas of fractures are the ribs, the upper arm (humerus), and the upper leg (femur).

If a patient is known to have metastases in the bone, it is sometimes a good idea to treat weak areas with radiation *before* they fracture. Side-effects of 'spot radiation' therapy to small areas are few and patients report prompt pain relief.

Chapter 31
Metastatic Bone Pain

Bone pain is one of the most difficult problems that is faced during the management of prostate cancer. At least 80% of patients with metastatic disease or progression of the disease after initial therapy will eventually have pain from bone metastases. Pain may be sudden and severe, or it may be a slowly-developing, constant ache. In both situations the patient's individual perspective on his disease, his emotional outlook, his life-long biases, and his family support will directly affect the severity and control of pain. Physicians are responsible for optimizing the quality of life of patients in the face of pain, and there are safe and effective means of achieving this.

Bone pain can be treated either by localized radiation, if only one or two spots are involved, or by some form of hormone or chemotherapy if the problem is more widespread. If a patient has never been treated for prostate cancer then the ideal approach is to castrate either surgically or medically. After hormone-withdrawal therapy, more than 80% of patients will have prompt and complete relief of the pain caused by bone metastases. The durability of the response is variable: on average, it lasts about two years. If a patient is at the terminal stages of his disease and has bone pain despite adequate hormone-withdrawal therapy, then comfort can be achieved by other means. **Analgesics** (pain killers), either non-narcotics or narcotics, alone or in combinations, will play an essential role in pain management. Patients with progressive, relapsing disease who receive narcotics to alleviate pain, should not be afraid of becoming addicted to the drugs (Demerol™, morphine). This is the type of pain that narcotics were designed for.

Physicians will tailor the analgesic regime to the person's needs. Analgesics can be combined with anti-inflammatory drugs or antihistamines, which often provide an additive pain-relieving effect while minimizing side-effects. Muscle relaxants or sedatives may also help. Patients should be on the look-out for side-effects from the analgesics such as nausea and vomiting, constipation or excessive fatigue. If these occur, or if the patient becomes tolerant to his level of medication, then an alternative drug should be started. When oral pain killers are no longer effective, then narcotics, given intramuscularly or intravenously, are helpful. Certain narcotics are available as rectal suppositories. Direct injection of the drug into the spinal canal may be considered in special circumstances; this is an 'in-hospital' procedure. Alternatively, a pump may be implanted under the skin with a tube leading into the spinal canal. A narcotic, such as morphine, can then be delivered continuously into the spinal canal by means of this pump.

If there are many metastases in the bony skeleton and the patient is suffering from generalized pain, radiation applied to half the body ('hemibody radiation') can be effective. This is quite a toxic form of treatment because so much of the bone marrow is irradiated that the patient's blood counts drop dramatically (most blood cells are produced by the bone marrow). It is also an uncommon form of treatment but nevertheless, there are numerous reports of patients obtaining significant pain relief within two to three days. The duration of the pain-relief response may be 4 to 6 months, often long enough to maintain an improved quality of life during the terminal stages.

Steroids, such as prednisone taken orally, or dexamethasone given intravenously, are important to the reduction of all types of cancer pain. It is estimated that 1/3 of patients with bone pain treated by prednisone obtain pain relief. In addition, steroids are known to improve the emotional state of the patient. While these are not the same types of steroids that athletes sometimes use, they are very powerful drugs, with potentially serious side-effects, therefore patients undergoing steroid therapy must be monitored closely.

Diphosphonates, drugs known to block the metabolic activity of normal bone cells, have been used to suppress metastatic cancer pain. They may prove to be valuable during the last few months of life, particularly if narcotics are no longer effective.

An interesting new agent is a radioactive material called **strontium**. It is injected intravenously and goes directly to areas of bone growth where it concentrates at the sites of cancer metastases and destroys many of the cells, shrinking the bone tumor and reducing pain. As it is very expensive, it has been reserved for patients who are in pain and at the terminal stages of their cancer.

Chemotherapy may be used for the patient with bone pain and hormone-independent cancer. If he is generally in good condition, but his cancer is progressing despite adequate hormone withdrawal, then his pain may lessen, even if only temporarily, in response to chemotherapy. Some centers report a decrease of pain medication requirements and sometimes even a total eradication of pain after treatment with chemotherapy. However, it is unlikely that chemotherapy will prolong life in such cases.

Lastly, if all of the above treatment methods fail to control pain, there are **surgical procedures** that can provide pain relief. These involve the neurosurgical cutting of the nerve fibers that conduct the pain. Severing the nerve can be done either as an open operation, or by injecting nerve-destroying medication *via* a needle passed through the skin under x-ray guidance. This treatment of pain is drastic but will provide the patient with pain relief and an alert state for his final days.

SECTION IX
LIVING WITH CANCER

Chapter 32

Impotence After Treatment

When a man who is sexually active undergoes treatment for prostate cancer, he must be prepared for the possibility of a decline of his sexual function. After radical prostatectomy a certain percentage of men will suffer partial or total loss of erections (**impotence**). However, **libido** (sexual desire) as well as the ability to experience orgasm without an erection may remain intact. Similarly, radiation therapy frequently leads to loss of erectile ability without a loss of libido. Surgical or medical castration, however, will cause both impotence and loss of libido because of the removal of the male hormone, testosterone, from the body.

Because it is possible for sexual function to return gradually after radiation treatments or radical surgery, most urologists tend to wait 6 to 12 months before instituting any form of therapy for impotence. The patient is assessed by a battery of tests including serum testosterone levels, kidney function and blood sugar. If these are all normal, and there are no underlying psychological or social interaction problems, then he can be considered for treatment.

Treatment options include stimulants of penile blood flow by oral medication or injection of a drug into the shaft of the penis (intracorporal injection), use of a vacuum inflation device and surgical insertion of a semi-rigid or inflatable penile prosthesis (artificial devices).

PENILE STIMULANTS

Erections are the result of increased blood flow to the penis. A drug known as yohimbine may be used to stimulate this blood flow. This drug has been found to be useful to men who have soft erections and some anxiety related to their ability to perform.

Since 1982, several drugs have become available that can be injected into the the penis to stimulate an erection. Known as vasoactive agents, these drugs lead to improved blood flow and retention of blood within the penis, resulting in a natural erection. The erection lasts anywhere from several minutes to several hours, depending on one's sensitivity to the drug. The drugs currently used are papaverine, phentolamine and prostaglandin (these may be mixed together to increase potency). They are *self-administered* by inserting a fine needle through the skin of the penis. The injection is relatively painless, although some practice is necessary to overcome the initial inhibitions. The man who becomes impotent following radical prostatectomy or radiation therapy will respond well to this form of therapy. Orgasm and sensation will be close to normal, however there will be no ejaculate since the sources of fluid (the prostate and seminal vesicles) had been removed by the surgery.

After a transurethral resection of the prostate (not radical prostatectomy), it is very rare to suffer loss of erections. However, an inability to ejaculate normally is common. This is because the bladder neck, the junction of bladder and prostate, has been damaged and the fluid ejects backward into the bladder rather than out the penis (fig 33). This is known as **retrograde ejaculation** and is not dangerous but it does create infertility, which is usually not an issue for the prostate cancer age group.

VACUUM DEVICES

If a patient is unhappy with penile injections, or is unable to tolerate them, there are alternatives. Vacuum therapy is based on the premise that impotence results from inadequate blood flow into the penis or from the inability to retain blood within the erectile tissue. Commercially-available vacuum therapy devices are noninvasive and act by creating a vacuum that generates blood flow into the penis. The blood is retained in the penis by a simple retention ring placed at the base of the penis once the erection has been obtained. Men who master this technique are very comfortable and satisfied with it because the resulting erection is quite natural in size and feel (although the ring can be irritating to some). This technique is generally safe, but should be avoided by patients who have blood disorders or penile abnormalities; and only used cautiously by patients who are on anti-coagulant medication. Before ruling out the possibility of using this technique, an individual should inspect the device and watch some demonstration tapes.

PENILE PROSTHESES

A popular form of therapy for lack of erection involves the implantation of prostheses (artificial devices) into the penis. Penile prostheses, which have helped thousands of men resume normal sexual intercourse, are available in semi-rigid and flexible, or inflatable formats.

The semi-rigid rods are implanted into the penis and produce a state of permanent erection. The penis remains flexible and may be positioned close to the body for concealment. The inflatable penile prostheses are more sophisticated and allow the man to determine when he has an erection. Inflatable prostheses are made up of several components. They have two cylinders that are implanted into the shaft of the penis, a balloon-like reservoir placed under the abdominal muscles, and a pump located in the scrotum (fig 45). None of the components can be seen once they are implanted and the prosthesis is quite easy to operate. By simply squeezing the pump in the scrotum, fluid is transferred from the reservoir into the cylinders to create an erection. When a release valve on the pump is pressed the fluid returns to the reservoir and the penis becomes soft again. The penis never feels perfectly normal with an inflatable prosthesis in place, but it is readily concealable.

Before deciding on the type of prosthesis, it is important for a man to discuss all his concerns and fears openly with both his physician and his sexual partner. The risks of prosthetic surgery are quite low but they do include the possibilities of pain, infection and rejection of the artificial device. Also, the inflatable prostheses may develop fluid leaks or pump

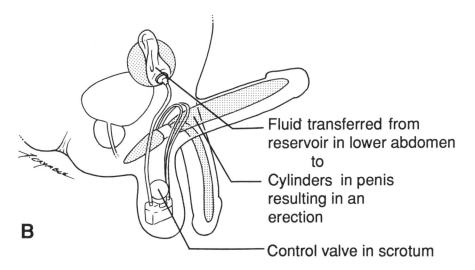

Fluid transferred from reservoir in lower abdomen to Cylinders in penis resulting in an erection

Control valve in scrotum

B

Figure 45. Components of inflatable penile prosthesis.

malfunctions. Fortunately, however, such problems are not common and the need to re-operate to repair the pump should happen in less than 10% of prosthesis cases.

Studies have shown that patients who have artificial prostheses and accept that the erection is never exactly the same as the one nature gave them, react well to sexual activity after surgery. As mentioned with the injectable drugs, ejaculation does not take place, but orgasm does, though it may be less intense.

SEXUAL ACTIVITY AND QUALITY OF LIFE

When a man learns that he has a malignancy, his first thought is survival. Treatment can cure prostate cancer in the early stages and control it in the later stages. Unfortunately, treatment often affects sexual activity and with it the quality of life of many patients. Even though a man has a prostate cancer, the treatment of which will leave him with reduced libido and increased anxieties, he need not ignore the fact that he still has a partner with positive sexual feelings who wants to maintain a satisfying relationship. Any of the means described above will enable him to do this. Because men tend to be uncomfortable talking about their lack of sexuality or sexual prowess, many communities provide discussion groups which help to deal with this problem. These discussion groups are led by urologists, and sex counsellors are available to help men understand and accept their impotence, and to provide them with support and treatment.

Finally, it is a common myth that sexual intercourse can spread cancer to one's partner. This is *not true* and should never be a source of anxiety for a couple.

Chapter 33

Urinary Incontinence After Treatment

CAUSES OF URINARY INCONTINENCE

Involuntary leakage of urine, after any form of prostate operation, is not a pleasant phenomenon, but knowing that it may happen, and that it will be transient or can be treated, makes it easier to deal with. Before undergoing surgery, a man should ask his urologist about the chances of incontinence in his particular case and also about the surgeon's preferences and biases with respect to postoperative management of the incontinence. As with the problem of impotence after treatment, an individual should feel free to obtain a **second opinion** so that he feels comfortable with the treatment approach.

The normal male has several mechanisms for controlling urination. These include the ring of muscle (sphincter) around the bladder neck (junction of bladder and prostate), muscle fibers in the prostate itself, and a voluntary muscle which is what one uses to consciously stop or start the urine stream (fig 37). Many patients who have an enlargement of the prostate, with or without a cancer, will find that they have an urge to void urine frequently. This is usually due to an irritable bladder muscle and inadequate emptying of the bladder. After the obstructing prostate gland is removed the irritability will disappear, but it may take several months. Similarly, after radical prostate surgery a patient may notice an urgent and frequent need to void not only during the day but also at night. Radiation, too, causes increased bladder irritability, but this usually disappears within a few weeks or months.

Occasionally, incontinence may be the result of direct invasion of the sphincter muscles by a large prostate malignancy, rendering the sphincter muscles incompetent. This situation may improve after hormone-withdrawal treatments.

A few patients develop incontinence after transurethral resection of the prostate. When a prostate is large, most of the urinary control depends on the prostate and the bladder neck mechanism. When this tissue is removed, as in a transurethral resection, the urinary control falls back on the voluntary sphincter and involuntary muscles that are left intact after surgery. Initially,

133

these muscles may be overwhelmed by their sudden, new responsibility and it may take some time for their strength to return to adequate levels. Occasionally, transurethral resection of the prostate may damage the sphincters. This is unusual, but can be managed by any of the techniques outlined below.

Following external radiation, incontinence occurs in less than 10% of cases. When it occurs it is most likely due to irritation and uncontrolled bladder contractions with or without some injury to the normal tissues of the sphincter. As the bladder irritability subsides, the incontinence improves.

Almost all patients have some degree of urine leakage after a radical prostatectomy. Eventually, however, 95% will regain near-total control or be left with only a minor degree of stress incontinence. This means the loss of a few drops of urine with change of position, coughing, sneezing, lifting heavy weights, or other sudden 'stresses.' All of these movements cause an increased abdominal pressure which in turn, is transmitted to the bladder. The rapid rise of bladder pressure is too much for the sphincter to withstand and some urine leaks out. At one year after surgery, about 5% to 10% of patients will continue to have significant **stress incontinence**. Continuous, total incontinence (as opposed to stress incontinence) occurs in less than 5% of cases.

CORRECTION OF URINARY INCONTINENCE

After prostate surgery, whether it be a transurethral prostatectomy or a radical prostatectomy, when the catheter is removed from a man's bladder, he should not despair if he has some urgency to urinate or some stress incontinence. A positive outlook should be retained since the problem is almost always transient. Initially, the patient should begin to exercise his voluntary urethral sphincter muscle. This is done by a technique known as **Kegel's exercises**. One concentrates on squeezing the muscles in the area of the anus. This squeezing action stimulates the same nerves that control the muscles used to hold back urine. Repeating this muscular action for several minutes every hour will help return control of urination. To remind one to do these exercises, it is useful to develop 'cues' by doing them during radio or television commercials, or at every red light while driving.

In the early postoperative period one should avoid using urine collection devices (*eg* condom catheter) on the penis as they may irritate the skin of the penis. They may also become a 'crutch' because they keep the clothing dry and make it easy to forget to do exercises or take medication. Adult diapers are a better alternative: these have been modified over the past few years and the currently available materials absorb urine extremely well so that there is very little odor. If the leakage is minimal, pads or folded tissues placed in the underwear are often sufficient.

If the incontinence continues to be a problem and is thought to be due to an overactive bladder muscle, then specific medications can be taken to counteract this. These drugs have side-effects including a dry mouth, blurred vision and constipation. They work well, however, on the bladder muscle and are worth considering for a short trial.

Several forms of surgical correction are available for urinary incontinence. The least invasive, most recent and, as yet unproven method involves the injection of a synthetic paste (teflon) or of a natural protein called collagen into the tissues around the urethra near the bladder. The injected material passively occludes the urethra and resists the increased abdominal pressures which are transmitted to the bladder during physical stress.

More established and more effective treatment involves implantation of an artificial sphincter device to control leakage (fig 46). The device is implanted through two incisions. A cuff is placed around the urinary channel behind the scrotum. This cuff is connected to a balloon reservoir of fluid which is implanted just under the muscles of the abdomen and to a control valve which is placed in the scrotum. In its natural state, the fluid is in the cuff compressing the urethra, thereby blocking both voluntary and involuntary urination. When a man wants to urinate he simply squeezes the bulb of the pump in the scrotum which transfers the fluid from the cuff around the urethra to the reservoir balloon. This opens the urinary channel so that urine can flow freely. Within 60 to 90 seconds the fluid automatically flows back to the cuff and continence is once again restored. This device does require an open operation for insertion, but the recuperation time is short, only one or two days in hospital. Recent refinements in the construction of the device have led to a very low mechanical failure rate. With all prosthetic devices there is a risk of infection or rejection and this applies to the artificial sphincter as well. Overall, however, the device works extremely well and is reliable.

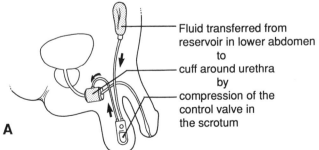

Fluid transferred from
reservoir in lower abdomen
to
cuff around urethra
by
compression of the
control valve in
the scrotum

A

Figure 46. Components of the artificial sphincter device.

Chapter 34

Living with a Cancer Diagnosis

Although every cancer patient and every family member is unique, the road each must travel is well-worn by the millions of others that have come before. It is a journey marked by hope and despair, courage and fear, humor and anger, and constant uncertainty. While the body undergoes tests and treatments, the mind searches for its own way of coping. This section is dedicated to the emotional effects of the diagnosis and treatment of cancer - the side of cancer that neither surgery, nor chemotherapy, nor radiation can treat.

IS THERE A 'RIGHT WAY' TO FEEL AFTER RECEIVING A CANCER DIAGNOSIS?

Many people are concerned that the thoughts and feelings that they experience following a diagnosis of cancer are somehow abnormal or crazy and that there must be a 'right' way to feel. This couldn't be further from the truth. There is *no one* way to feel. Reactions to the diagnosis can span the full range of human emotion: anger, anxiety, uncertainty, hopelessness, helplessness, depression, a feeling of isolation, vulnerability, relief that there really is something wrong, and even guilt that one has somehow contributed to the development of his or her own disease, or delayed in bringing it to a doctor's attention.

It is important to realize that the initial reaction to the diagnosis will be followed by other feelings. It is an emotional process or journey that occurs. Just as we go through a series of 'stages' in accepting the loss of a loved one, we pass through a number of emotional levels on our way to acceptance of the diagnosis of cancer. First, there is often disbelief in the diagnosis, denial that it is true, and anger at being 'singled-out.' Finally, there is acceptance. Why we go through these stages is difficult to know. Psychologists postulate that the time required to progress from disbelief to acceptance may offer protection by creating time and space for adjustment.

136

"I felt shocked... numb... like it wasn't real. I don't think I really felt anything for a week and then I felt betrayed." "I decided that the doctors had made a mistake and that any minute someone would come out and say it had all been an unfortunate mistake."

Expressions of very strong emotion are to be expected and they may range from anger and bitterness to frank hostility which may be directed at anyone and anything.

"I was angry at everyone... God in particular... I hadn't done anything to deserve this.""I just wish that they had let me die. They should just have let me go to sleep and never wake up after the operation."

As the initial anger and anxiety begin to settle, denial becomes the prominent response. Denial is a defense against fear and early on helps to maintain emotional equilibrium. The patient believes that the diagnosis is wrong, that it doesn't have anything to do with him. It is not uncommon to hear people comment "I think he's in denial" as if there may be something unusual and potentially dangerous about this reaction. In fact, some degree of denial is normal and it is probably necessary to protect oneself and to maintain the hope needed to participate in daily life. However, it is important to recognize that denial is healthy only as long as it does not interfere with seeking medical care or participating in appropriate treatment.

"At some level I had to distance myself from the reality of the cancer in order to listen to the information that I was being given. I had to think that this was about someone else... It really protected me but it drove my wife crazy."

Fortunately, most people will emerge from the storm of emotions to reach a point of equilibrium and acceptance, although transient periods of regression are common. At what point this acceptance finally occurs in any one individual is difficult to predict.

"The cancer made me realize how precious life is. I used to waste time... now I use every minute." "Cancer... a rare opportunity... I discovered how special my sister was."

COPING WITH CANCER

Every person has a unique tool-box of coping strategies that have been accumulated over a lifetime. Most will find what they need to meet the challenge of cancer.

> "How did I cope initially? I don't know, really... I guess I did the things that I've done in other tough situations... I turned to my family and friends, then the nurses and doctors."

There are as many coping skills as there are people. Seeking information, turning to family and friends for support, developing a partnership with the health care team, maintaining hope and learning stress management techniques are all means by which the coping 'mindset' develops

Seeking Information

Appropriate information can help to allay some of the anxiety and fear associated with the unknown. The type and amount required varies with the wants and needs of the individual and family. Generally, people want to know about diagnostic tests, treatment plan (purpose, expected results, side effects, length of time and scheduling), and prognosis. Essential, but often neglected information concerns how the disease and treatment are likely to affect the person's daily life. Your local chapter of the Cancer Society is an excellent place to look for this kind of help. Most local chapters of the Society provide booklets, seminars, stress management training, and self-help groups for individuals with cancer and their families. A list of Cancer Society chapters are included at the end of this book in Appendix C.

Of course, your doctor is a critical provider of information pertinent to your particular problem. When attending your physician or other members of the health care team, don't be afraid to ask questions. They will be expecting it. Prepare a list, otherwise you may forget important points that you have been wondering about. Write down the answers and, if you wish, take someone along to help you remember what was said. The early phase of diagnosis and treatment can be somewhat of a daze and having a spare pair of ears around is very helpful.

Telling Others

In most cases, your family and close friends will learn sooner or later that you have cancer. It is usually best to disclose the information yourself, according to your own schedule. Confiding fears and hopes is an important part of developing the coping mindset, and in the long run it is easier than trying to conceal these important feelings.

There are some situations in which it may be best not to tell. Family members that are too old, too young, or too emotionally fragile may have difficulty accepting or understanding the situation. However, it is quite extraordinary how most people can summon the courage to adapt to the reality of illness and the possibility of death, even when it involves someone that they love very much.

Sometimes family members are the first to learn the diagnosis and they will occasionally attempt to shield the patient from the information in what is usually a misguided attempt to protect that person from the pain of knowing. In certain instances, such as when the patient is extremely old or young, or very ill and cannot understand, this is sensible. In the vast majority of cases, however, it is better for the patient to know. Otherwise, important relationships that should be strengthened become strained and artificial as loving family members and friends try to skirt the issue and discuss only superficial matters. Worse than that, in almost all such cases, the individual finds out anyway, all too often at an inopportune and harmful moment and probably from someone who doesn't even know him well. Don't let this happen. Given the truth about the situation, sensitively presented, the patient is permitted the opportunity to evolve naturally toward the point of acceptance, and can set his or her mind on important priorities. Everyone is owed that much.

Telling young children that their parent or sibling has cancer can be especially troubling. The goal in telling children that someone in the family has cancer is to give them opportunities to ask questions about the disease and to express their feelings about it. While we all wish to shield our children from pain, it is better that they experience pain in a way that they understand and can talk about with their parents, than to cope with sorrow on their own in forms that become embellished by their imagination. Moreover, if they are denied knowledge of the cause of why there has been great disruption in the family, they may become confused and hurt and mistakenly believe that that they are responsible.

Support Groups

In many cities there are support groups consisting of people living with cancer and trained professionals who manage the sessions. The professionals provide a forum where the person with cancer can be open about his thoughts and feelings, and can discover that these are normal and acceptable. Other members of the group often suggest alternative ways to deal with difficult issues, ways that have helped them. Seeing others who are coping with similar situations can aid in identifying solutions to problems which seem overwhelming initially. In addition, membership in a formal group may give the cancer patient a means to overcome a feeling of helplessness by offering assistance to others.

"Although my family was supportive, I felt as if they couldn't possibly understand what it was like for me. I needed to talk to someone else who had cancer. That doesn't mean that you shouldn't talk to your family but it's different when you talk to another survivor. In the Living with Cancer Group, I found that I could give something back... which was very important as it was the first time in a long time that I felt useful."

Developing a Partnership with the Health Care Team

At one time, patients and families were considered to be silent members of the health care team, if indeed they were considered team members at all. Today, people with cancer are encouraged to take an active role in treatment planning.

The first step in developing a partnership with the health care team is to *know who the players are* and what each one has to offer. This can be a challenging task as, over the course of time, there are often many different specialists involved in the care of the patient and family. It is important to identify one team member who will serve as the **leader**, usually the family doctor, the urologist, the **oncologist** (cancer specialist) or a specialist nurse. It doesn't matter who assumes the role as long as he or she is able to relate to the patient and family and will be there for the duration. This person should be available at regular intervals, or when required, to listen to concerns, to direct questions to the appropriate professionals, and to serve as guide and support.

The second important step is to *participate in decision-making about treatment.* Although this may seem impossible because of what appears to be an overwhelming amount of information that needs to be taken into account, a skilled physician should be able to simplify the facts so that two or three alternatives can be presented at any stage of treatment.

"I had a life threatening illness and I was being asked whether I wanted this treatment or that treatment. I felt that my life was on the line if I made the wrong decision. I didn't know whether

140

or not I wanted that responsibility. Then I realized that I knew me better than anyone else and that knowledge would be helpful in making a good decision."

No matter how complex your problem may seem, your specialist is expected to be able to help you through the decision-making processes by providing you with the framework of the 'big picture,' thereby simplifying decisions. His or her ability to explain that is essential to provide you with the information you need to participate. Once a few of the initial choices are made based on such information, you will have some time to seek additional sources and pursue the educational process that will support you later on.

Participating in decision-making means listening to the options, identifying their advantages and disadvantages, comparing them to your own values and aspirations and those of your family. Some patients will want to discuss all of the options, perhaps seeking a **second opinion** before making an informed decision with or without their families. Others might be uncomfortable making the final decision, but can still participate by clarifying their values and wishes so that the final recommendations for treatment can be tailored to their needs.

The third step in developing a partnership with the health care team is to *participate in the treatment plan* - managing the side effects of the treatment, reporting changes in condition, attending follow-up appointments, providing team members with feedback about how things are progressing, and using the services and supports that are available.

A Note About Changing Doctors

Clearly, excellent communication between patient and doctor is critically important to the successful adaptation of the patient to diagnosis and treatment. Unfortunately, some physicians never learn to speak comfortably with their patients or families, and in the name of some sort of professionalism let people down by not being 'there' for them when tough choices have to be made. Although such physicians may appear to be abrupt, aloof and uncaring, they are usually not. Nevertheless, if this problem creates a barrier, ask your family doctor to refer you to someone else. Remember, you almost always have a choice in who treats you so don't be afraid to find someone that you are comfortable with. Keep in mind, however, that a decision to change physicians should be based on reality and not on a quest to find a doctor who will promise a cure and guarantee to relieve all your fears.

141

When Friends Don't Call

Lost and strained friendships are a particularly painful aspect of dealing with cancer. Friends do not call for a variety of reasons. For most, it is out of a feeling that they will have so little to say that will help, and a fear that they might instead say something hurtful. Others may be afraid that they will not be able to respond appropriately to your change of appearance, or they are fearful of facing the possibility of your death and the eventuality of their own.

> "I see that my friends don't know how to talk to me, and they shy away from me."

None of these reasons have anything to do with your friends' view of your worth and, indeed, some may be suffering themselves from the loss of their normal relationship with you. If you believe that it is discomfort that is keeping a particular friend from visiting, you might try a phone call to dissolve the barrier. This often reassures them that you are still the same person that they liked before, and that you understand their difficulty. However, don't expect to change or enlighten everyone. We all have our own emotional capabilities and timetables and some people will not be comforted sufficiently for them to maintain the relationship as it was before.

Maintaining Hope

Hope is a crucial tool for cancer patients and their families. It is the internal resource that permits one to accept or better tolerate the stresses associated with diagnosis and treatment. Loss of hope reduces one's ability to adjust to the situation.

Hope means different things to different people and tends to change over time depending on the stage of the disease and treatment:

> "There is always hope, it just changes. First you hope that you don't have cancer, then you hope that the cancer is curable or at least treatable. Then you hope for time and finally, you hope for a good going. If you lose hope you give up."

Maintaining and nurturing hope is a strategy that can allay anxiety, depression and fear. Nurturing hope means focusing on the present and what is immediately ahead, rather than on the future or the past, neither of which can be changed. While this reorientation of focus can be difficult in our future-oriented society, it can help manage the daily challenges of cancer treatment.

Hope can be responsive to the behavior of others. Those around the individual and family must be not only aware of the hopes that are held but also should attempt to share in them or to shape them into more attainable goals. Family members and friends can support the idea that there is nothing wrong with being hopeful and they should not classify hope as false.

> "Be prepared for the worst but hope for the best. There is no such thing as false hope. Everyday I hope for a miracle, but that doesn't stop me from continuing in my treatment nor would it stop me from acceptance if my treatment is no longer working. If you took my hope away I don't know if I would want to continue..."

Hope is not based on false optimism or benign reassurance, but is built on the belief that better days or moments can come in spite of the situation.

SECTION IX
APPENDICES

APPENDIX A:
Case Scenarios

Each of the following cases illustrates a different clinical situation: one or more may provide useful insights.

NOT ALL SYMPTOMS MEAN CANCER

A forty-nine year old man notices slowing of his urinary stream and an increased urgency to void in the morning. He is also troubled by getting up once at night to urinate but does not have any burning, bleeding or pain with urination. He is concerned that he has a cancer and visits his physician. The only abnormality found is a minimal enlargement of the prostate, which feels otherwise soft and smooth on finger examination. He is told that he has early signs of prostate enlargement but no evidence of cancer or infection and is asked to return on an annual basis for a digital examination of the prostate and review of his symptoms. No further investigations or treatment are undertaken.

> *Author's note: In our concern to impart awareness of cancer symptoms, we often fail to mention that the most common cause of urinary problems is not from cancer at all, but from benign disorders of the prostate such as infections and BPH. However, the diagnosis must be confirmed by careful examination lest cancer be overlooked, thereby delaying necessary treatment. In this case, the patient's youth and the obvious rectal findings "fit" with the diagnosis of a benign problem.*

AN ABNORMAL PSA TEST RESULT

A fifty-nine year old man in good health discusses his concern regarding prostate cancer with his family practitioner. The patient's father died of prostate cancer at age sixty-eight and he has heard that he is also at risk of developing the same problem. The doctor confirms the patient's impression and arranges for a PSA blood test.

Five days later, the family practitioner contacts the patient and tells him that the test result is elevated to '10', which is 'slightly' abnormal. He refers the man to a specialist who examines the prostate by rectal examination and finds it to be normal in size and consistency. A transrectal ultrasound does not reveal any abnormalities but because of the elevated PSA and the family history of prostate cancer the specialist takes some directed biopsies of the gland. Two of these biopsies contain malignant tissue. A subsequent search for metastases included a bone scan and tumor markers. All of these were normal and the patient was booked to undergo a radical retropubic prostatectomy for treatment of stage B2 cancer.

At the time of surgery, his pelvic lymph nodes were examined carefully and no cancer was found. The tumor was felt to be confined to the prostate and therefore it was removed in its entirety. When the pathologist later examined the removed tissue he confirmed that cancer was confined to the prostate gland. This man thus had a pathological stage B prostate cancer and he remains well.

> *Author's note: In this man, even with a normal rectal examination, the elevated PSA and positive family history are enough to raise a suspicion of cancer. The PSA can be marginally increased (4 to 10) by benign prostatic enlargement but the onus is on the physician to rule out cancer in the presence of an elevated PSA. When the PSA is higher than 10, even with no symptoms and an absolutely normal physical examination, one-third of men will be harbouring a cancer in their prostate.*

AN OCCULT CANCER

An apparently healthy sixty year-old man notices painless bleeding on urination. It lasts for only one day. He is referred to an urologist whose examination reveals a prostate that is moderately enlarged but feels benign. An intravenous pyelogram shows normally functioning kidneys and an ultrasound fails to reveal any abnormalities of the kidneys, bladder or prostate. Blood tests, including PSA, are all within normal limits The urologist recommends that the patient undergo a cystoscopic examination of the bladder.

By means of the cystoscopy the urologist learns that the prostate gland is moderately enlarged and has some dilated blood vessels on its surface. The bladder is thickened but contains no signs of cancerous growths, stones or other abnormalities. During a transurethral resection of the prostate, a core of tissue is removed and carefully examined by the pathologist. She reports that 1% to 2% of the specimen contains a well-differentiated prostate cancer.

The patient is sent for further testing. A bone scan shows no abnormality. He is told by his urologist that he has a clinical stage A1 cancer which has a low chance of progressing to a higher stage. Because of his relative youth, however, his urologist suggests that more tissue be removed from his prostate and examined under the microscope. This is done six weeks after the initial operation and another 15% of the tissue is found to contain cancer.

The urologist informs him that his cancer is stage A2 and recommends a radical prostatectomy. The alternative options include radical radiation therapy, hormone-withdrawal therapy or no further treatment. After discussions with his wife and family and careful consideration of the consequences, the man opts for the radical surgery, which is carried out uneventfully. As a first step in the operation, the lymph nodes are removed and examined microscopically and no cancer is found. The prostate is removed in its entirety and the bladder reconnected to the urethra.

While subsequently examining the entire removed prostate gland, the pathologist finds areas of residual cancer, though apparently none has spread outside of the gland. The patient has pathological stage A2 prostate cancer which, completely removed, has an excellent outlook for survival. He recovers fully, though his sexual function is diminished for 5 to 6 months after his operation. Gradually his erections return to normal and he becomes fully continent of urine. He now returns semi-annually for a digital examination of the prostate area and measurement of his serum prostate specific antigen. There is only a 10% chance that his cancer will return either within the pelvis or at a metastatic site.

Author's note: This patient had symptoms related to enlargement of the prostate gland and was found to have an occult cancer when the transurethral resection was performed. He underwent a repeat, 'staging transurethral resection'. An alternative is to take multiple samples of tissue by ultrasound guided biopsy. Some urologists would recommend going directly to radical prostatectomy in such a case because of the high probability of residual cancer and eventual disease progression. The treatment of stage A remains controversial. For now, all cases must be individualized.

146

A WORRISOME PROSTATE NODULE

A fifty-five year-old man undergoes a physical examination after applying for a new life insurance policy. The examining physician finds a small nodule in the man's prostate gland and refers him to an urologist. The specialist feels that the nodule could be a cancer. A biopsy confirms the presence of a well-differentiated cancer. Transrectal ultrasound shows no other abnormalities within the prostate, and biopsies taken from other "normal-feeling" parts of the gland are benign. The bone scan and PSA are normal. Because of the man's relative youth and the well localized cancer, the urologist recommends a radical prostatectomy. He agrees to undergo surgery. During the operation, it is found that the lymph nodes are clear and the entire prostate is removed. Despite the benign preoperative biopsies, the pathologist finds many cancerous areas in the "normal-feeling" portion of the prostate, ranging in grade from well- to moderately well-differentiated. There is no evidence of cancer spreading outside of the capsule into the surgical margins or seminal vesicles. The patient makes an uneventful recovery and is followed-up on an annual basis with a digital examination of the prostate area, and measurement of the serum prostate specific antigen.

> *Author's note: This man's cancer involves more of the prostate gland than was appreciated by preoperative testing. It is not uncommon for a cancer to be "understaged" as when multiple areas of the prostate contain cancer, though only a single nodule can be palpable. As long as all the "margins" are clear one is hopeful that it was removed 'just in time.'*

THERAPEUTIC FAILURE

Digital examination of a sixty seven year-old man discloses an enlarged and rocky-hard prostate. He is referred to an urologist who does a prostate biopsy and confirms the diagnosis of a stage C, moderately well-differentiated cancer. It is recommended that the patient undergo a pelvic lymph node dissection for staging purposes. At the time of surgery the pelvic lymph nodes are all found to be clear of cancer. Subsequently, a six week course of radiation therapy is beamed at the prostate gland. During the weeks of therapy, the patient gradually develops reduced energy, transient diarrhea, and urinary urgency. Three months later, however, his urinary stream is excellent and his bowels regular. His energy level is good and he feels well.

The patient is seen by his family physician every three months during the next two years. Although it initially seems to his physician that the prostate is shrinking, it gradually begins to increase in size again. Two years after completion of his radiation therapy, the patient is sent back to the urologist for reassessment. A repeat biopsy of the prostate shows that there is still active cancer within the gland. The serum PSA is twice normal and a bone scan shows two new hot spots in the spinal column which were not present two years earlier. The patient is now considered to have stage D2 cancer. Treatment is begun with a combination of monthly LHRH agonist injections and a daily antiandrogen tablet. Within a few weeks the PSA returns to normal.

> *Author's note: Radiation therapy can cure localized, stage C cancer in approximately 60% of cases. In the remainder the cancer will gradually resume its growth and 'recur.' In the above scenario, the patient may have had microscopic metastases at the time of diagnosis, metastases that did not become apparent until two years later. This is the type of patient who might have profited from adjuvant hormone-withdrawal therapy. Unfortunately, there is no way of identifying these patients at the time of primary treatment. Currently, there is insufficient evidence to support the concept that treating all stage C patients with hormone-withdrawal therapy will result in greater benefit than potential harm.*

PATHOLOGIC FRACTURE

A seventy eight year-old man has a minor fall and fractures his right hip. X-rays of the area suggest a pathologic fracture (a fracture through a metastasis) plus other metastases within the pelvic bone. Examination of his prostate shows that it is enlarged and firm, but it does not feel cancerous. Because of his age and the x-ray findings, a PSA test is done which comes back sharply elevated, suggesting the presence of prostate cancer. To establish the diagnosis, a transrectal ultrasound of the prostate gland is done and biopsies are taken from suspicious areas. These show malignant cells.

It is recommended to the patient that he undergo some form of hormone-withdrawal treatment for metastatic prostate cancer. The first treatment offered is surgical castration. He declines this, preferring to consider medical alternatives for at least a few months. He is started on monthly LHRH analogue injections and an oral antiandrogen drug which he takes twice daily. This rapidly lowers his serum testosterone levels and he begins to feel quite well. The back-aches that had bothered him prior to the fall disappear. His hip gradually heals although he requires a single dose of radiation therapy to the area of the fracture. He continues on the medication for six months and then undergoes surgical removal of the testicles under local anesthetic. He tolerates this procedure well and stops the medications. He continues to live reasonably well.

    Author's note: Patients with advanced prostate cancer often respond rapidly and dramatically to hormone-withdrawal therapy. It is not unusual to see men throw away their crutches within a few days of commencing therapy. Unfortunately, in 90% of cases this response will only last a couple of years.

APPENDIX B:
Radical Prostatectomy - A Patient's Perspective

(The author is grateful to Mr. Robert Bacon for writing this essay and permitting it to be published as part of this book.)

"Well I'm afraid that you do have a spot on your prostate gland. It's malignant and you will have to have either radical prostate surgery or radiation and hormone-withdrawal therapy."

Oh God! I couldn't believe it. The little nodule had been discovered in the course of a standard check-up and I had been assured that it was almost certainly benign. "You are just too healthy and strong for it to be a problem, but just in case..." Well it wasn't benign and I was one of those one in 10 guys who are going to get prostate cancer. "60% of all those men who come in to see us about their prostate pain have waited too long. You don't feel any pain as a rule until the cancer has spread to the surrounding lymph nodes and then it's too late." Such comforting words! I hung on to the fact that I had felt no discomfort and so I was going to be OK, but that night while my wife was sleeping, I stared at the blackness and gave in to my terror. My father, a reformed heavy smoker, had died from lung cancer, my grandfather had succumbed to stomach cancer, and now me?

How could I relay this to my 90 year old mother alone in her little house, 6000 miles away, in England? Well, she wasn't going to know about it, that was for sure and neither would any of my family still living there. There was nothing they could do about it except worry themselves sick. For them, 'cancer' was synonymous with 'death.' The problem of relaying the news to my children turned out to be not so difficult. The four older ones, 28 down to 20, were very supportive and confident that their indestructible old dad (I'm 55) would be fine, and my wife and I soft-pedalled the news to the two still in the house: teenage girls have enough on their minds without the extra burden of a sick dad.

It was strange to see how my colleagues at school accepted the news.

Many were very sympathetic and scared enough to go immediately to have their prostates checked, but many others absolutely ignored me as though I were a leper. "If I don't talk to you, then I'm not going to get it."

I did not feel comfortable with the off-handedness of my first surgeon and the hospital where he worked looked really grubby and disorganized. Discouraged, I went to see a second urologist. His hospital confirmed the previous diagnosis and so I had to face up to it. "There are 4 stages of cancer," he said, "A through D; A and B are operable, but C and D are too late. "You have..." (a long pause) "...a B2, it's touch and go." He suggested a program of anti-hormone tablets that would shrink the cancer and confine it to the prostate and, when the cancer was as small as it could be, then he would operate and remove the gland and the tumor.

I found that I needed to have my wife accompany me to the monthly meetings with the surgeon, as I was not able to digest much of what he said. In the first few months, the lack of pain and the remoteness of surgery (it was going to be a 6 month hormone treatment), made me feel that the doctor was talking about someone else and then as the fateful day approached, that, together with the bone-numbing tiredness that the hormone pills induced, made me hardly able to pay attention.

The prolonged hormone treatment had a variety of effects on me, both physical and mental. I was first given my 'cancer drug number' which allowed me free treatment at the 'Cancer Clinic' with what would otherwise have been expensive drugs. This number depressed me, it seemed akin to the hood and bell of the medieval leper, or the tattoo given to the inmates at Dachau and Auschwitz. I was 'unclean,' avoid me. Whenever I went to the clinic to have the prescription renewed, I would look into the room where the 'cancer support' group met. Everyone there seemed hollow-cheeked and ready for the morgue. I would never be caught dead in there, I said to myself. I grew to hate that place. I also found myself reading the obituary column in the newspaper. How many had died from cancer? How old were they? How many of them were men? My wife, who is a librarian, could not bring herself to read about prostate cancer and though my surgeon had advised that I read to learn more about the disease, I could not do it at first. Like Red China, if you ignore it, maybe it will go away.

The first physical symptom I felt was a loss of desire to make love to my wife. It began a few weeks after the start of the hormone treatment. Our sex life had been gorgeous and frequent. I would still delight in watching her undress and be naked in our room at night. She in no way tried to be provocative, but was just the same natural woman as always. But I felt no sexual response and more importantly, I felt no humiliation at being unable to be aroused. It was as if I had no sexual organ at all. My wife was wonderful

151

throughout this whole time and never gave me the slightest feeling that she was dissatisfied or frustrated.

About 4 months into the treatment, it was in the shower that I first noticed how tender my nipples had become. As I was soaping myself one morning, it felt as if I had been stung by a wasp. It became so that during the last 6 weeks, I could not bear to have my wife lean her head on my chest. Throughout this whole time, the ever-present fatigue was gradually dominating everything. The slightest thing became an enormous effort. I am an extremely active man, I cycle to and from school every day, coach a highly unsuccessful rugby team there, and I faithfully use our exercycle each morning, but during the last two months of the treatment I was out of it by midday. Luckily for me, the school where I teach had given me the whole fall term off in readiness for my October operation. I couldn't have faced the kids productively. I also became very sensitive to heat and cold and noticed that after my workout on the exercycle I was hardly sweating and my sweat didn't have the old rankness I was used to. I later learned from my GP that the hormones I was using were similar to the ones produced by expectant mothers. So there I was, 6'5", 240 lbs, bearded and pregnant!

Despite all the side-effects, which are inevitably unpleasant, I was determined to keep a positive attitude. I told myself that the side-effects proved that the pills were working and so they must be attacking the cancer in the hoped-for manner. I never gave in to the possibility that I was not going to pull through and I was given enormous support in this by the many friends and colleagues I had gathered over the years. Close friends and people dimly remembered would call me up and tell me how their father or brother had suffered from the same problem 10 or 15 years ago and had successfully recovered. Many of my friends, some of them doctors, got me started on the power of positive thinking. I read books in which patients had made miraculous recoveries from what seemed to be hopeless situations. They were all written by doctors of traditional western medicine and these authors all claimed that it was the patients' indomitable spirit and their determination to get well that had cured them. I engaged in 'visualization' techniques with the help of a colleague of mine, and I imagined the cancer in my body and demanded that it respond to the treatment and I told my body to heal itself. I was helped in this by the knowledge that a surgeon friend of mine used this technique on some of her own patients. As a teacher for some 20 years, I knew how vitally important a positive and determined attitude was. I have had many students who were not particularly gifted, but whose determination to learn to the best of their abilities had vaulted them past students with far greater natural talent, but without the courage to use it.

However, I must admit that in the last week, I did become a bit despondent and frightened. I wondered if the outward signs of the pills' effects on me were not being mirrored within. Six months is a long time for a cancer to spread and grow if unchecked, particularly a borderline one. All this was despite my surgeon's assurances that the tumors (Oh God! More than 1?) were shrinking and softening properly and that my cancer count was well below 'the top of my boots.' Throughout all of this period, I had become acutely aware of the pain and anguish that my wife was suffering. It was compounded by the fact that she got very little attention. It was always, "How is Bob?" and seldom, "How are you?"

The preparatory day before my operation passed as in a dream. Various nurses came and went. IVs were stuck in my arm, some foul-tasting fluid was forced upon me to completely clean out my digestive tract. Apparently there is a possibility that the intestines may be punctured during the operation and they obviously must be devoid of any material likely to cause infection. This experience was, without doubt, the most unpleasant of my whole hospital stay. Drinking about a gallon of liquid that tastes as if it had been previously used to preserve dog-fish in some high school laboratory is not my idea of epicurean delights. This misery was compounded when the nurse instructed me that she wanted to see my bowel movements, to check on their increasing clarity and purity. Having finally decided that my innards were squeaky clean, she then unceremoniously shaved those parts near and dear to me and left me to contemplate the next 12 hours.

I remember being totally relaxed and at ease. I felt that I had come through the 6 months pretty well, that there was a great deal that I had to live for, that I was being prayed for and supported by so many wonderful people. I had great confidence in my surgeon's ability to cure me and the hospital seemed to be both efficient and caring. In the late evening, I phoned my wife for mutual reassurance and her strength added to my feeling of well-being.

This was still with me when I was woken the next day and I felt rather excited at the prospect of what was going to happen to me. I was absolutely confident that this was the beginning of the end of my tiredness, my sore nipples, my hot and cold flushes and that the old rampant man so well known to myself and my wife would soon be reemerging.

Waiting outside the operating room doors, the two nurses at the head of my bed were extremely gentle and attentive. They assured me that I was in the best possible hands, that I would not feel any pain and that everything was going to be all right. As it turned out, they were right! The operation was a complete success. The surgical team came in to my room to congratulate me and through the haze I could see my wife and oldest daughter beaming through their tears, and the place was a mass of flowers. Apparently, my borderline situation made it necessary for the surgeon to 'cut pretty deep,' but his delight at the results was very evident.

The week of recuperation in hospital was interesting. I soon learned how hard the nursing profession worked and how difficult their task often was. Many patients seemed to think that their particular needs should be dealt with immediately and that 'thank-you' did not appear to be a very frequently used word. However, the nurses all gave the impression that they understood the pain and fear that many of the patients suffered and made all kinds of allowances. They were great with helping me, helping me to exercise my legs to prevent clots and making sure I did the deep breathing and coughing exercises needed to prevent pneumonia. They all kept emphasizing how essential a positive attitude towards the situation was. Any dignity that I thought that I might possess quickly disappeared in the urology ward. More pretty young ladies sponged off my genitals in the first few days of recovery than had done so in my previous 20 years. When I first checked in to the hospital, the head nurse had asked me if I objected to a female nurse shaving me and generally caring for postoperative needs. Apparently most men do object to this. I have a hunch that women do not often get this option in similar circumstances. It was then that I began to understand why some women have felt less than charitably toward the predominantly male medical industry. Their Pap tests, obstetric and routine gynecologic investigations are generally done by men, who, with the best will in the world, cannot appreciate how their patients really feel.

My overall feelings were those of relief and gratitude to the family, friends and professionals who had helped me make it through. When the man with the scythe thinks about making a serious visit in your direction, it has a way of focusing your attention on things that matter. Had I not been diagnosed with cancer, I would never have learned the affection so many people had for me. I had been having a rather difficult time with one of my children, but she wrote me the most wonderful and loving card, and all of our previous problems have disappeared and now we are the best of friends again. Neither of us can understand what the fuss had been all about. Somewhat of a price to pay for such peace, I suppose, but now that it is all over and I am out of danger, I feel better for having gone through it. It does seem a pity though, that for the most part, we don't want to cross our emotional bridges until they are burning out beneath us. I was also happy that I had changed hospitals and surgeons. I am sure that the first ones that I went to were perfectly sound, but they were not comfortable for me. We shop around for houses and cars, so why not for doctors? Our bodies are more important to us than to anyone else, surely.

And so, one month after the operation, I walk about 6 to 8 blocks every day. I have a slight urinary infection and my incontinence has all but vanished. I find it difficult to sit for very long periods and my libido has shown little sign of returning. I have tried to be patient with myself. The initial improvement is very noticeable, but the minor problems of abdominal discomfort and general suppleness, do not seem to get much better with the passing days. It will just take time, 6 months I'm told, before a complete recovery. I have learned how precious life and loved ones are. I hope that I never forget.

Author's note: This man was treated with anti-androgens before radical prostatectomy in the hope that this would result in 'down-staging' his clinical stage B2 cancer. Fortunately, this was successful and all the cancer was removed by the surgery. It should be emphasized that this approach is not general practice. In fact, this concept of down-staging is currently under scientific evaluation.

APPENDIX C:

Support and Service Organizations

CANADIAN CANCER SOCIETY

The Canadian Cancer Society is a national, voluntary organization which provides information, assistance and direction for patients with cancer. The society's goal is to optimize the quality of life of patients and their families by means of a wide variety of social, emotional and psychological support programs.

NATIONAL OFFICE
77 Bloor St. West, Suite 1702
Toronto, ON M5S 3A1
(416)961-7223

BRITISH COLUMBIA AND YUKON
565 West 10th Avenue
Vancouver, BC V5Z 4J4
(604)872-4400

ALBERTA AND
NORTHWEST TERRITORIES
2424 - 4th St. SW, Suite 200
Calgary, AB T2S 2T4
(403)228-4487

SASKATCHEWAN
2445 - 13th Avenue, Suite 201
Regina, SK S4P 0W1
(306)757-4260

MANITOBA
193 Sherbrook St.
Winnipeg, MB R3C 2B7
(204)774-7483

ONTARIO
1639 Yonge St.
Toronto, ON M4T 2W6
(416)488-5400

QUEBEC
5151 boul. de l'Assomption
Montreal, PQ H1T 4A9
(514)255-5151

NEW BRUNSWICK
P.O. Box 2089
Saint John, NB E2L 3T5
(506)634-3180

PRINCE EDWARD ISLAND
P.O. Box 115, 131 Water St.
Charlottetown, PE C1A 1A8
(902)566-4007

NOVA SCOTIA
201 Roy Building, 1657 Barrington St.
Halifax, NS B3J 2A1
(902)423-6183

NEWFOUNDLAND AND LABRADOR
P.O. Box 8921
St. John's, NF A1B 3R9
(709)753-6520

CANCER CENTRES AND CLINICS

Cancer centres provide chemotherapy and radiation treatment, as well as information and support programs.

BRITISH COLUMBIA

British Columbia Cancer Agency - Vancouver Clinic
600 West 10th Avenue
Vancouver, BC V5Z 4E6
(604)877-6000

The Victoria Cancer Clinic
1900 Fort St.
Victoria, BC V8R 1J8
(604)595-9228

Interior Cancer Clinic c/o Royal Inland Hospital
311 Columbia St.
Kamloops, BC V2C 2T1
(604)374-5111

ALBERTA

Cross Cancer Institute
11560 University Avenue
Edmonton, AB T6G 0T2
(403)432-8771

Tom Baker Cancer Centre
1331 - 29 St. N.W.
Calgary, AB T2N 4N2
(403)270-1711

Lethbridge Cancer Clinic
1802 - 9 Avenue South
Lethbridge, AB T1J 1W5
(403)329-0633

SASKATCHEWAN

Saskatchewan Cancer Clinic
University Hospital
Saskatoon, SK S7N 0X8
(306)966-2662

Allan Blair Memorial Clinic
4101 Dewdney Avenue
Regina, SK S4T 7T1
(306)359-2333

MANITOBA

St. Boniface Hospital
409 Tache Avenue
Winnipeg, MB R2H 2A6
(204)233-8563

Manitoba Cancer Treatment and Research Foundation
100 Olivia St.
Winnipeg, MB R3E 0V9
(204)237-2559

ONTARIO

The Ontario Cancer Foundation Hamilton Centre
711 Concession St.
Hamilton, ON L8V 1C3
(416)397-9495

The Ontario Cancer Foundation Kingston Centre
King St. W.
Kingston, ON K7L 2V7
(613)544-2630

The Ontario Cancer Foundation North East Program
41 Ramsey Lake Road
Sudbury, ON R3E 5J1

The Ontario Cancer Foundation Ottawa Centre - Civic Hospital Division
190 Melrose Avenue
Ottawa, ON K1Y 4K7
(613)725-6300

The Ontario Cancer Foundation London Centre
391 South St.
London, ON N6A 4G5
(519)697-9890

The Ontario Cancer Foundation Thunder Bay Centre
290 Munro St.
Thunder Bay, ON P7A 7T1
(807)345-1425

The Ontario Cancer Foundation Toronto-Bayview Centre
2075 Bayview Avenue
Toronto, ON
(416)488-5801

The Ontario Cancer Foundation Windsor Centre
2220 Kildare Road
Windsor, ON N8W 2X3
(519)253-5253

The Ontario Cancer Institute
Princess Margaret Hospital
  500 Sherbourne St.
  Toronto, ON M4X 1K9
  (416)924-0671

QUEBEC

Centre hospitalier universitaire de Sherbrooke
  3001 - 12th Avenue N.
  Sherbrooke, PQ J1H 5N4
  (819)566-5555

Hopital general de Montreal
  1650 Cedar Avenue
  Montreal, PQ H3G 1A4
  (514)937-6011

Hopital general juif de Montreal
  3755 chemin de la Cote Sainte-Catherine
  Montreal, PQ H3T 1E2
  (514)340-8222

Hopital Hotel-Dieu de Chicoutimi
  Avenue Saint Vallier, C.P. 1006
  Chicoutimi, PQ G7H 5H6
  (418)549-2195

Hopital Hotel-Dieu de Montreal
  3840 rue Saint Urbain
  Montreal PQ H2W 1T8
  (514)843-2611

Hopital Hotel-Dieu de Quebec
  11 cote du Palais
  Quebec, PQ G1R 2J6
  (418)691-5151

Hopital Maisonneuve Rosemont
  5415 boulevard de l'Assomption
  Montreal, PQ H1T 2M4
  (514)252-3400

Hopital Notre-Dame
  1560 est, rue Sherbrooke
  Montreal, PQ H2L 4K8
  (514)876-6421

Hopital Royal Victoria
  687 avenue des pins ouest
  Montreal, PQ H3A 1A1
  (514)842-1231

NEW BRUNSWICK

Department of Radiation
Oncology & Nuclear Medicine
  Saint John Regional Hospital, P.O. Box 2100
  Saint John, NB E2L 4L2
  (506)648-6884

PRINCE EDWARD ISLAND

Oncology Division
  Department of Health and Social Services
  P.O. Box 2000
  Charlottetown, PE C1A 7P1
  (902)566-6027

NOVA SCOTIA

Halifax Cancer Centre
  5820 University Avenue
  Halifax, NS B3H 1V7
  (506)429-4200

NEWFOUNDLAND

St. John's Cancer Clinic
  General Hospital, Health Sciences Centre
  Prince Philip Drive
  St. John's, NF A1B 3V6
  (709)737-6300

UNITED STATES

ALABAMA

University of Alabama at Birmingham
Comprehensive Cancer Center
  University Station, Birmingham, AL 35294
  (205)934-5077

ARIZONA

Arizona Cancer Center,
  University of Arizona Health Sciences Center
  1501 N. Campbell Avbenue,
  Tucson, AZ 85724
  (602)626-6044

CALIFORNIA

City of Hope Medical Center
  1500 East Duarte Road,
  Duarte CA 91010
  (818)359-8111

Loma Linda University Medical Center
  11234 Anderson St.,
  Loma Linda, California 92354
  (714)796-7311

Donald P. Locker Cancer Center
  1414 South Hope St.,
  Los Angeles, California 90015
  (213)742-5634

UCLA Jonsson Comprehensive Cancer Center
  10-145 Factor, 10833 LeConte Ave.,
  Los Angeles, CA
  (213)206-2805

University of Southern California
Comprehensive Cancer Center
  1- 441 Eastlake Ave.,
  Los Angeles, CA 90033
  (213)224-6600

Santa Clara Valley Medical Center
  751 South Bascom Ave.,
  San Jose, CA 95128
  (408)299-5635

Stanford University Medical Center
  Stanford, CA 94305
  (415)497-7311

COLORADO

AMC Cancer Research Center and Hospital
  1600 Pierce St.,
  Denver, CO 80214
  (303)233 6501

CONNECTICUT

Yale Comprehensive Cancer Center
  333 Cedar St.,
  New Haven, CT 06510
  (203)785-4095

DISTRICT OF COLUMBIA

Vincent T. Lombardi Cancer Research Center
  Georgetown University Medical Center
  3800 Reservoir Road, NW
  Washington, DC
  (202)625-7721

FLORIDA

University of Florida College of Medicine
  J. Hillis Miller Health Center,
  Gainseville, FL 32610
  (904)392-3261

Papanicolaou Comprehensive Cancer Center,
  University of Miami, School of Medicine
  Miami, FL
  (305)584-4800

H. Lee Moffitt Cancer Center &
Research Institute,
  University of South Florida
  12902 Magnolia Drive,
  Tampa, FL 33682-0179
  (813)972-4673

GEORGIA

Regional Cancer Center - St. Joseph's Hospital
  5665 Peachtree Dunwoody Road, N.E.
  Atlanta, GA 30342
  (404)851-7110

Winship Cancer Center,
  Emory University School of Medicine
  1327 Clifton Road,
  Atlanta, GA 30322
  (404)248-5180

Enoch Callaway Cancer Clinic
  111 Medical Drive,
  Lagrange, GA 30240
  (404)882-1411

HAWAII

Cancer Center of Hawaii
  1236 Lauhala St.,
  Honolulu, HI 96813
  (808)548-8415

IDAHO

Mountain States Tumor Institute
  151 East Bannock St.,
  Boise, ID 83712-6297
  (208)386-2711

ILLINOIS

Northwestern University Cancer Center
  303 East Chicago Avenue,
  McGaw Pavilion 8250,
  Chicago, IL 60611
  (312)908-5250

University of Chicago Cancer Research Center
  5841 S. Maryland Avenue, Box 44,
  Chicago, IL 60637
  (312)702-6180

KANSAS

University of Kansas Cancer Center
  University of Kansas Medical Center,
  Rainbow Blvd. at 39th St.,
  Kansas City, KS 66103
  (913)588-4700

KENTUCKY

Lucille Parker Markey Cancer Center
  800 Rose St., University of Kentucky
  Lexington, KY 40536
  (606)233-6541

Cancer Center - University of Louisville
  Health Sciences Center, P.O. Box 35260,
  Louisville, KY 40232
  (502)588-5245

James Graham Brown Cancer Center
  529 South Jackson St.,
  University of Louisville,
  Louisville, KY 40292
  (502)588-6905

LOUISIANA

Touro Infirmary
1401 Foucher St.,
New Orleans, LA 70115
(504)897-7011

MARYLAND

Johns Hopkins Oncology Center
600 North Wolfe St.,
Baltimore, MD 21205
(301)955-8818

National Cancer Institute
9000 Rockville Pike,
Bethesda, MD 20892
(301)496-4000

MASSACHUSETTS

Boston University Cancer Research Center
Boston Univ., Med. Center,
80 East Concord St.,
Boston, MS 02118
(617)247-6075

Brigham and Women's Hospital
75 Francis St.,
Boston MS 02115
(617)732-5542

Dana-Farber Cancer Institute
44 Binney St.,
Boston, MS 02115
(617)732-3000

New England Deaconess Hospital
185 Pilgrim Road,
Boston, MS 02215
(617)732-7000

Veteran's Administration Hospital
150 South Huntington Avenue,
Boston, MS 02130
(716)232-9500

Saint Vincent Hospital
25 Winthrop St.,
Worcester, MS 01604
(617)798-1234

MICHIGAN

Henry Ford Hospital
2799 West Grand Boulevard,
Detroit, MI 48202
(313)876-1852

Meyer L. Prentis Comprehensive Cancer Center of Metropolitan Detroit
3990 John R Suite 505 Hudson,
Detroit, MI 48201
(313)745-4700

MINNESOTA

University of Minnesota - Masonic Cancer Center
University of Minnesota Medical School
Univeristy Hospitals, Box 286,
Minneapolis, MN 55455
(612)373-4303

Veteran's Administration Medical Center - Cancer Research Division
54th St. and 48th Ave S,
Minneapolis, MN 55417
(612)725-6767

Mayo Comprehensive Cancer Center
200 First St. SW,
Rochester, MN 55905
(507)284-2511

MISSOURI

Ellis Fischel State Cancer Center
115 Business Loop 70 West,
Columbia, MS
(314)875-2100

St. Louis University Medical Center
1402 S. Grand Blvd.,
St. Louis, MS 63104
(314)664-9800

NEBRASKA

Bishop Clarkson Memorial Hospital
44th and Dewey Avenue, PO Box 3328,
Omaha, NE 68103
(402)559-2000

NEW HAMPSHIRE

Norris Cotton Cancer Center of the Dartmouth Hitchcock Medical Center
2 Maynard St.,
Hanover, NH 03756
(603)646-5505

NEW MEXICO

University of New Mexico - Cancer Research and Treatment Center
900 Camino de Salud NE,
Albuquerque, NM 87131
(505)277-2151

NEW YORK

Albany Regional Cancer Center
317 South Manning Blvd., Suite 330,
Albany, NY 12208
(518)489-2607

Our Lady of Lourdes Memorial Hospital,
Regional Cancer Center
169 Riverside Drive,
Binghampton, NY 13905
(607)798-5431

Roswell Park Memorial Institute
666 Elm St.,
Buffalo, NY 14263
(716)845-2300

Beth Israel Medical Center
First Avenue at 16th St.,
New York, NY 10003
(212)420-2000

Columbia University Comprehensive Cancer
Center
701 West 168 St.,
New York, NY 10032
(212)305-6905

Downstate Medical Center
450 Clarkson Avenue,
New York, NY 11203
(212)270-1000

Memorial Sloan Kettering Cancer Center
1275 York Avenue,
New York, NY 10021
(212)794-7000

Nassau County Medical Center
2201 Hemptstead Turnpike, East Meadow,
New York, NY 1554
(516)542-0123

NORTH CAROLINA

Lineberger Cancer Research Center of the
University of North Carolina
CB No. 7295,
Chapel Hill, NC 17599-7295
(919)966-3036

Duke Comprehensive Cancer Center
Box 3814, 227 Jones Building,
Duke University Medial Center,
Durham, NC 27710
(919)684-2282

OHIO

Ohio State University Comprehensive Cancer
Center
Suite 302, OSUCCC, 410 W. 12th Ave.,
Columbus, OH 43210
(614)422-5022

PENNSYLVANIA

Fox Chase Cancer Center
7701 Burholme Avenue,
Philadelphia, PA 19111
(215)728 6900

Hahnemann University
Broad and Vine Sts.,
Philadelphia, PA 19102
(215)448-8417

University of Pennsylvania Cancer Center
3400 Spruce St., 6 Penn Tower Hotel,
Philadelphia, PA 19104- 4385
(215)662-7979

RHODE ISLAND

Roger Williams Clinical Cancer Research
center
825 Chalkstone Avenue,
Providence, RI 02908
(401)456-2070

SOUTH CAROLINA

Cancer Treatment Center
701 Grove Road,
Greenville, SC 29605
(803)242-7070

TENNESSEE

University of Tennessee, Memphis, Cancer
Center
800 Madison Avenue,
Memphis, TN 38163
(901)528-5150

Vanderbilt Cancer Research and Treatment
Center
D-3300, 21st Avenue South,
Nashville, TN 37232
(615)322 3354

TEXAS

Charles A. Sammons Cancer Center
Baylor University Medical Center,
3500 Gaston Avenue,
Dallas, TX 75246
(214)820-3472

Wadley Institutes of Molecular Medicine
9000 Harry Hines Blvd.,
Dallas, TX 75235
(214)350-9011

University of Texas Medical Branch, Cancer
Center
G. 104 Microbiology Building, J20,
Galveston, TX 77550
(409)761-2981

The University of Texas M.D. Anderson Cancer
Center
1515 Holcombe Boulevard,
Houston, TX 77030
(713)792-2121

VERMONT

Vermont Regional Cancer Center
1 South Prospect St.,
Burlington, VT 05401
(802)656-4414

VIRGINIA

Massey Cancer Center
401 College St., Box 37,
Richmond, VA 23298-0001
(804)786-0448

WASHINGTON

Fred Hutchinson Cancer Research Center
1124 Columbia St.,
Seattle, WA 98104
(206)467-5000

**Marian Cheney Olrogg
Regional Oncology Center**
Tacoma General Hospital,
315 South K St.,
Tacoma, WA 98405
(206)597-6964

WISCONSIN

Wisconsin Clinical Cancer Center
600 Highland Avenue,
Madison, WI 53792
(608)263-8600

Index

163

chief resident 69, 101
chronic prostatitis 17
clinical stage 48
clone 3
cobalt radiation equipment 105
collagen 135
colorectum 21, 27
complication 76, 94, 98, 102
computerized axial tomography 44
condom catheter 134
constipation 126
continence 15, 75, 80
contraindication 76
cost of screening 56
creatinine 33
CT scan 44, 50, 62, 123, 125
cure 12, 58, 115, 118, 141
cyclophosphamide 65
cyproterone acetate 112
cystoscopy 38, 123

D

daughter cells 1, 3
delirium tremens 91
Demerol™ 126
DES 110
dexamethasone 127
diabetes 102
diagnosis 136
diarrhea 106, 113
dietary fat 27
diethylstilboestrol 110
differentiation system 13
digital rectal examination 30, 41, 48, 55
diphosphonate 117, 127
DNA 2, 104
drain 80, 88
dysplasia 84

E

early stage 12, 48
ejaculation 75, 130
ejaculatory ducts 15
ejaculatory fluid 15

electrolytes 33
emphysema 97, 103
endometrioid cancer 25
endotracheal tube 86
environment 27
erection 109, 129
Estracyt 116
estrogen 65, 110, 112, 116, 121
eunuch 28
exploratory surgery 41, 46
external beam radiation 105, 107

F

fatigue 112, 126
female hormone 110, 116
fever 96
fluid retention 111
fluorouracil 65
flutamide 112
Foley catheter 80, 99
follow-up 93
frequency 17, 29

G

gamma camera 41
general anesthetic 72, 86
genetic 2, 3, 104
glands 23
GnRH 110
gold grains 107
goserelin 113
grade 12, 13, 14, 46, 50, 57
growth factors 65, 117
gynecomastia 110, 112, 113

H

hard lump 30
heart attack 2, 98, 111, 112
heart disease 102, 112
hematoma 89
hematuria 20, 24, 29
hemibody radiation 127
hemoglobin 32
hemorrhage 9, 88, 124

165

R

radiation therapy 57, 58, 60, 61, 62, 63, 64, 104, 119, 121, 123, 125, 147, 129, 130, 136, 157
radical perineal prostatectomy 76
radical retropubic prostatectomy 58, 60, 61, 62, 76, 77, 129, 130
radioactive 41
radioactive 'seeds' 107
radioimmunoassay 33
radiotherapist 107
radium 107
rads 104
recovery room 87, 89
rectum 21, 99, 106, 107
recurrence 93
red blood cells 24, 32
relapse 65, 93, 117
remission 58
resection margin 85
resectoscope 73, 74
resident 69, 101
residual urine 18
retention 29
retrograde ejaculation 75, 130
retroperitoneum 46
reversing 88
RIA 33
rush section 77

S

salvage prostatectomy 58
sarcoma 25
scar 91
screening 53, 55
secondary site 7
secondary therapy 120, 121
seminal vesicles 15, 81
sensitivity 55
serum tumor markers 22
sexual function 28, 64, 65, 75, 110, 113, 114, 129, 132
shellfish 44

shortness of breath 112
side-effects 64, 65, 114, 116, 117, 119, 121, 126, 127, 135
signs 29, 32
Smoking 27, 77, 97, 102, 103
specificity 55
specimen 81
sphincter 134
spinal anesthetic 72, 109
spinal cord 113, 124
spinal cord compression 125
stage 11, 14, 41, 48, 57, 84, 142, 151
Stage A 48, 60, 61, 76, 146
stage B 48, 62
stage C 63
stage D 50, 64, 65
staging 61
staples 91
steroids 127
stitches 91
stomach upset 113
stress incontinence 134
stroke 102, 111
strontium 117, 127
suprapubic catheter 123
Suramin 65
surgical castration (see *castration*)
surgical castration 114
surgical judgment 95, 101
surgical pain 89
surgical residents 69, 101
swelling 46
symptoms 29, 32, 69

T

tattoo 106
technetium-99m diphosphonate 41
testicles (see *castration*)
testosterone 15, 20, 26, 28, 64, 65, 109, 110, 112, 113, 114, 115, 116, 121, 129
testosterone surge 113
therapy 57
third space loss 90

tingling 125
tired 64
transfusion (see *blood transfusion*)
transitional cell carcinoma 25
transrectal ultrasound 22, 35, 37, 56
transurethral prostatectomy 58, 60, 61,
    72, 73, 74, 123
treatment options 57
treatment simulator 106
tumor 5
tumor markers 22, 33, 63
TURP (see *transurethral prostatectomy*)

U

ultrasound 37, 123
ultrasound guidance 35
ureter 16, 24, 40, 43, 99, 123
urethra 15, 18, 63, 81, 123
urgency 17, 29
urinalysis 32
urinary blockage 29
urinary control 15, 75, 80
urinary tract infection 32, 74, 97
urine culture 32
urine volume 90
urologist 34, 38, 141

V

vacuum therapy 130
vas deferens 15
vasectomy 27
vasoactive agents 130
visitors 92
visualization 152
vital signs 88
vomiting 113, 126

W

Walsh's procedure 78
weakness 64, 107, 125
weakening of bones 122, 125
well-differentiated 13, 14, 46, 48, 50, 60,
    63
white blood cells 24, 32
wound infection 46, 97

X

x-ray 41, 106

Y

yohimbine 129

Z

zinc 28